SCIATICA SOLUTIONS

Also by Loren Fishman, MD, and Carol Ardman

BACK PAIN: HOW TO DIAGNOSE AND CURE
LOW BACK PAIN AND SCIATICA

CURE BACK PAIN WITH YOGA

SCIATICA SOLUTIONS

*Diagnosis, Treatment, and Cure for
Spinal and Piriformis Problems*

Loren Fishman, MD,
and Carol Ardman

W. W. NORTON & COMPANY
NEW YORK   LONDON

For information about permission to reproduce selections from this book, write to
Permissions, W. W. Norton & Company, Inc., 500 Fifth Avenue, New York, NY 10110

Manufacturing by RR Donnelley, Bloomsburg
Book design by Lovedog Studio
Production manager: Julia Druskin

Library of Congress Cataloging-in-Publication Data

Fishman, Loren.
  Sciatica solutions : diagnosis, treatment, and cure for spinal and piriformis problems
/ Loren Fishman, and Carol Ardman. — 1st ed.
     p. cm.
  Includes bibliographical references.
  ISBN-13: 978-0-393-05834-5 (hardcover)
  ISBN-10: 0-393-05834-4 (hardcover)
  1. Sciatica—Treatment. I. Ardman, Carol. II. Title.
RC420.F57 2006
616.8'56—dc22

                                                        2006009865

ISBN 978-0-393-33041-0 pbk.

W. W. Norton & Company, Inc., 500 Fifth Avenue, New York, N.Y. 10110
www.wwnorton.com

W. W. Norton & Company Ltd., Castle House, 75/76 Wells Street, London W1T 3QT

  3 4 5 6 7 8 9 0

This book is dedicated to Edward F. Delagi, MD, esteemed teacher, fellow fisherman, and friend, who approached electrodiagnosis as an extension of the physical examination, making possible a logical approach to sciatica.

ACKNOWLEDGMENTS

WE WOULD LIKE TO THANK Tova Ovadia, PT, for her experience and advice through the years, and for her caring for all patients, especially those with sciatica and piriformis syndrome. To Stephanie Leaf, PT, our gratitude for editorial suggestions and oversight.

For invaluable assistance with the surgery section of this book, we are indebted to Franco Cerebona, Chief of Spinal Surgery, Department of Orthopaedic Surgery, at St. Vincent's Hospital in New York City.

It was our luck to find Robert Finkbeiner, who has done intelligent, accurate drawings for this book, and has offered creative solutions to technical problems.

We are grateful to Evan Carver for his responsiveness and dependable good humor. Thank you to our patient editor, Jill Bialosky, and to Ellen Levine, our friend and agent.

NOTE TO READERS

THIS BOOK is not a substitute for medical advice and assistance. The judgment of individual therapists and physicians who know you is essential. Although the information in this book may help you identify the cause of your sciatica, only a doctor or other professional can provide a definitive diagnosis.

CONTENTS

Part II
CONTROL and CURE

Part I

SCIATICA and PIRIFORMIS SYNDROME

Chapter I

DEFINING THE PROBLEM

HERE, IN SHORT FORM, is a classic story told to me in one variation or another by hundreds of intelligent, sensitive patients from every walk of life. After physical stress (including marathon sitting in a car or an office), after a fall or other accident, after lifting something extremely heavy, or sometimes for no apparent reason at all, they get a backache. The pain is severe enough and lasts long enough that they go to the doctor. Often pain and strange sensations radiate down the leg in searing, lightning-like shocks, or there is numbness or weakness in areas of the leg, or intense pain in the buttock. When that happens, the patient has sciatica.

Unfortunately a bout of sciatica is often a memorable experience. It's hard to forget something so unpleasant. If you have had sciatica, or if you have it now, don't despair of being able to cope. There is a great deal you can understand and do about this condition.

In the following pages we try to demystify this often confusing complaint, guide you in figuring out its cause, and give you tips about how to deal with it—medically and on your own. Sciatica has a way of wearing patients down, of making them feel defeated. We can assure you that there are many excellent methods for dealing with this problem. Clearly, the more you understand about it, the better off you'll be.

* * *

EVERY YEAR tens of millions of individuals experience back pain that causes them to seek medical attention. These people's pain translates into time and huge costs—lost days of work, lost activities and dollars. In 1998 alone, people with back pain spent $90.7 billion on their health care, and, as we all know, costs are always rising![1]

To some extent, the determinants of sciatica and low back pain are different.[2] Although back pain can be caused by a muscular or other problem, sciatica is not. Sciatica is almost without exception the result of a neurological problem in the back, or an entrapped nerve in the pelvis or buttock. Very rarely, other neurological conditions, such as multiple sclerosis or stroke, may account for it.

Sciatica and back pain overlap, but they are not always present together. Some people have back pain and sciatica. Some have sciatica without back pain, and some have back pain without sciatica. Sciatica, a special subcategory of problem that often accompanies back pain, is often lumped together with it, without regard to other symptoms and causes. That's a shame, because sciatica is widespread and deserves to be studied and acknowledged statistically and medically.

Digging deeply enough into the literature often reveals some estimates of its prevalence and possible treatments. Some studies have linked occupation, height, and time spent driving with sciatica as opposed to musculoskeletal or other types of back pain.[3] Although researchers haven't thoroughly analyzed back pain statistics by category of problems and symptoms, and more investigation is needed to discover how many individuals who have backache also have sciatica, a paper in the *Journal of Neurosurgery: Spine* did estimate that the prevalence of sciatica in the adult population of the United States is greater than 5 percent, and over a lifetime an individual has as high as a 40 percent probability of experiencing it.[4]

When it comes to piriformis syndrome—a compression of the sciatic nerve in the buttock and a frequent cause of sciatica—we have more information, but that information may not be conclusive. In 1983, an estimate came out of the Mayo Clinic that about 6 percent of the people who have sciatica have it because of piriformis syndrome.[5] According to that estimate, every year close to 5 million people in the United States have sciatica caused by nerve entrapment by the piriformis muscle. Research done in 2005 suggests that that number may be much higher.

A fairly recent study by recognized experts in the field found that 67 percent of their sciatica patients had no evidence of spine abnormalities on imaging studies, and that for them the common means of treating sciatica as a spine-originating symptom were not effective.[6] Under 20 percent of the 1.2 million sciatica-related MRIs revealed significant spinal problems, suggesting that piriformis syndrome may be quite common.

Writing in 1996, researchers from the Department of Neurosurgery at Johns Hopkins University admitted that they did not know how to care for the large group of patients who had sciatica without obvious spinal abnormalities, but they did not consider piriformis syndrome as a possible cause of these patients' pain. This conclusion was, and unfortunately still is, common.[7] In that same decade, some of the most prominent back pain specialists in the country defined sciatica as "symptoms and findings considered to be secondary to herniations of a lumbar disk."[8] Yet this does not take into account all the patients who have sciatica but no detectable problem in their spines.

WHAT SCIATIC PAIN FEELS LIKE

As I mentioned before, trauma, falls, overextending yourself physically, being cramped in an airplane or a car seat or elsewhere, and lifting something improperly are just some of the things that can result in sciatica. Still, I want to caution you: there's an old rule that doctors quote ironically, "post hoc, propter hoc." In other words, if B happened after A, it must be because A caused B. Put another way, you may have an automobile accident after turning on the car radio, but that doesn't mean that the two are related. Causes aside, there are a number of ways that problems with nerves—in this case, nerves in the back or buttocks—manifest themselves.

First of all, there's pain, which can be a dull ache, a sharp sting, electric-shock-like feelings, throbbing, or discomfort that comes and goes. It's always within your leg, along the course of the sciatic nerve and/or the territory that the sciatic nerve fibers serve on your skin.

Second, numbness occurs when the nerve impulses are unable to get through. Although numbness (which generally happens on the side of the calf, on the top or bottom of the foot, or on the heel or sole of the foot) seems an attractive alternative to pain, it may actually be a more important danger signal that the nervous system is unable to communicate warnings from the affected part of the leg back to the brain. Obviously, when you're numb, your insensitivity to pain may leave you open to injuring yourself without knowing it.

Parasthesias—strange sensations—are another manifestation of various types of nerve damage. Numbness is when you don't feel something that is there, such as sensation on the outside of your ankle or your foot, pressure on your calf, or fullness in your bladder. Parasthesias occur when you feel something that isn't there. So, you may experience the sensation of burning down the back of your thigh, though nothing is touching it. Electric-shock-like flashes, tingling, tightness, pins and needles, and the sensation that you have ants or other insects crawling on you also often appear when there is a problem along the course of the sciatic nerve.

Parasthesias may occur when communication between the central nervous system and the lower parts of the body is not halted but is disrupted enough that normal patterns are distorted and misread by the brain. Like the pain and numbness of sciatica, parasthesias are always located in the regions served by the sciatic nerve.

There are general similarities between sciatic pain, numbness, and parasthesias. All have their origins in the brain, spinal cord, or peripheral nervous system. All manifest themselves in the areas served by specific nerves—in this case the sciatic nerve. All have to do with problems in the conduction of nerve impulses.

Another hallmark of sciatica is weakness. Weakness isn't exactly a feeling, but you can feel it and it can be associated with sciatica, as can abnormally weak reflexes in the legs and feet. Nerve damage in the spinal cord can produce weakness in a specific pattern. Some of the most common manifestations of such nerve damage (more about this later; see page 23) are weakness in the back of the calf and difficulty walking on tiptoe, foot dragging or slapping, knees buckling, or difficulty rising from a sitting position.

Warning: If you have back pain and/or symptoms of sciatica and at the same time you suddenly experience incontinence of either bowel or bladder, you may be suffering from nerve fiber involvement called cauda equina syndrome. Although this condition is not fatal, it may be serious. You should see a physician or go to an emergency room immediately.

IS SCIATICA PERMANENT?

Sciatica is unpleasant. Sometimes it's debilitating. Often it seems as though it will never go away. The question of how long sciatica lasts is one that has been studied extensively over the years, and some of the conclusions are contradictory. However, in my experience sciatica usually does go away, with or without surgery. How quickly you can get rid of the pain, and how completely, is variable. The discomfort may recede with almost intolerable slowness, even taking years.[9] Yet many patients who have herniated disks find relief within 30 days. The very nature of sciatica is somewhat mysterious, even to the people who study it and treat it every day.

It is certain, however, that surgical and nonsurgical techniques are evolving, and the results for patients who have operations are improving steadily. On the other hand, waiting may be as effective as having surgery. One survey done by the Agency for Health Care Policy and Research (AHCPR) found that, ten years later, people who had had surgery and those who had not experienced almost the same degree of cure. In other words, whether or not you have surgery, you are likely to recover from a bout of sciatica—eventually. In the group studied by the AHCPR, the people who had the more serious conditions and the most severe pain helped select themselves for surgery. But just how often those people chose to have an operation and how often people suffering greatly refused surgery and found effective conservative measures hasn't been sorted out. Nor do we know how many not-so-awful cases chose surgery because they were frightened that their condition wouldn't improve without it, or for other reasons.

My experience suggests that 95 percent of sciatica patients who have seen me in my office at least twice have gotten substantial or complete relief.

The Maine Lumbar Spine Study, which has been publishing results of investigations into back pain since 1996, has tried to assess the difference in recovery between patients who have had various levels of treatment. The conclusions are far from definitive. In 1996, researchers analyzed baseline-interview questionnaire answers from 507 patients who had been treated surgically for sciatica caused by herniated disks and 232 patients who had not had surgery. After a year, the group that had surgery improved more than the group that did not have it. However, for patients who entered the study with relatively mild symptoms, the benefits of surgical and nonsurgical treatments were similar.

The same group of researchers assessed five-year outcomes for patients with sciatica caused by lumbar disk herniation and found that, of the 402 patients whose results were available, 63 percent of those who had surgery reported satisfaction with their current status, whereas 46 percent of those who didn't have an operation were not satisfied. Surgery seemed to bring the most relief early in the follow-up period, but again the difference between surgical and nonsurgical groups narrowed over the years.[10]

Later we'll discuss in more detail the pros and cons of surgery, injections, physical therapy, and other remedies. For now, it's important to say that there are several steps to take before you are faced with a decision about surgery.

Regardless of the precise details of your individual case, sciatica can be so severe that it keeps you in bed. Actually, at one time bed rest was the prescription for this condition. Today objective empirical work has shown that bed rest is not necessarily the best way to treat sciatica. I believe that being up and doing about 40 percent of what you usually do is the best way to deal with it.

A recent review of published studies about this question concluded that staying active in itself doesn't do much for low back pain patients and has even less of a beneficial effect on people with sciatica. But staying active isn't harmful, and prolonged bed rest can cause deconditioning and other problems. Lack of activity can weaken you generally, which is a possibly dangerous consequence of spending too much time in bed.[11] If I had to recommend a single treatment for low back pain and sciatica, it would be to stay active.[12] (See pages 159–70 for a more thorough discussion of yoga and exercises that will help maintain a healthy back.)

WHAT SCIATICA IS

Experiencing something unpleasant in addition to back pain is a complicating factor in many of my patients' stories. In some cases the back pain has lessened or even disappeared, only to be accompanied by or replaced by other, equally or even more uncomfortable problems, including numbness, weakness, hot or cold or tingling or burning sensations in the legs, or pain down the thigh or the side of the leg. The patients with extra discomfort—a large subgroup of the millions with back pain—have sciatica, or nerve pain.

This nerve pain is nothing new. Our ancestors had it, and so did their ancestors. Sciatica is common enough and painful enough to have been noticed and documented since the fifth century BC, when it was described by Greek physicians. The Romans associated sciatica with gout, osseous tuberculosis of the bone, hip dislocation, and polio. In the fourth century AD, physicians believed that sciatica was characterized in part by a "strong, severe pain emanating from the lower back and radiating into the buttocks, perineum and even the popliteal fossa [a lozenge-shaped space at the back of the knee joint], the calf, foot and toes." Some ancient remedies—bed rest, massage, heat, and passive range-of-motion exercises—are treatments we still use with some success today. But in Roman times patients suffering from intense sciatica were also likely to be subjected to leeches, bloodletting, and the laying on of hot coals.[13]

Our understanding of sciatica has been slow to evolve over the millennia. There was a great leap forward, however, in the early twentieth century, with the work of William Mixter and Joseph Barr. In 1934 these two doctors published a groundbreaking article in the *New England Journal of Medicine* that changed public perception of the nature of sciatica by establishing and confirming the link between pressure on nerve fibers generated by intervertebral disk problems and sciatica.[14]

Now, thanks in part to Mixter and Barr, sciatica is broadly defined as pain in the lower back, buttocks, hips, or adjacent areas, including skin; it also refers to pain along the course of the sciatic nerve, which is the largest nerve in the body (*Merriam-Webster's Medical Dictionary*). The usual places to feel sciatica are in the back of the thigh, down the back of the leg, on the outside of the calf, on the side of the foot, and in the heel. Although pain farther up in the back is real and legitimate and deserves attention and treatment—and may be associated with damage to nerve fibers that may or may not be part of the sciatic nerve—any pain you feel above the buttocks isn't sciatica.

Many patients who come to me know that they have sciatica, or nerve pain. But they have a basic misunderstanding of the nature of their condition. They believe that the *cause* of their pain is sciatica. Not so.

Your doctor may listen to what you have to say about what's bothering you, examine you, and say, "You have sciatica." This could give the impression that you have a diagnosis for your problem. But sciatica is a symptom, not a cause of pain or other discomfort. Your doctor may be able to tell you that you have sciatica, but not be able to pinpoint the exact cause of your discomfort. Sciatica often needs attention from medical professionals, but so do its causes.

Chapter II

CAUSES AND TYPES
OF SCIATIC-TYPE PAIN

SEVEN CAUSES OF SCIATICA

1. Compression of the sciatic nerve by a herniated disk in the back.
2. Spinal stenosis (narrowing of the spinal column).
3. Spondylosis (degenerative spinal osteoarthritis, often associated with aging).
4. Nerve entrapment. The most common example is piriformis syndrome, in which a muscle in the buttock is causing not only muscular pain but is pressing against the sciatic nerve and causing sciatica. A recent article found that two-thirds of non-disk sciatica was caused by nerve entrapment in the buttock.
5. Inflammation and swelling from any other type of arthritis, sprains, joint slippage, or possibly infection.
6. Vascular problems. In the late stages of pregnancy, due to increased blood volume in the spine, the fixed space inside the spinal cord may narrow, compressing nerves and causing sciatica; for those with a condition called "pseudo sciatica," or intermittent claudication, poor blood supply in the legs can mimic sciatica after short walks.

The compression, inflammation, reflex mechanism, or entrapment problems briefly described above are associated with the nerve fibers that travel through the spine, exit it, and pass down through the body to the lower extremities. These fibers from the sciatic nerve and other nerve fibers behind the sacrum travel down the legs and into the feet. The referred pain mechanisms include pathways going through the same points but originating above the spinal cord, often in the brain.

7. Central mechanisms. Stroke or cerebral hemorrhage or multiple sclerosis can, on occasion, result in pain in the sciatic distribution. Referred pain is an especially relevant central mechanism of pain. It is a reaction by the central nervous system to a condition having nothing to do with the sciatic nerve, but the nervous system reacts in such a way as to cause pain to be felt along the sciatic nerve. People are discovering additional referred sources of sciatica and other pain, including complex regional pain syndrome (CRPS), also known as reflex sympathetic dystrophy syndrome (RSD). It is a condition that exhibits a group of typical symptoms, including pain (often a "burning" pain), tenderness, and swelling of an extremity. These symptoms are associated with varying degrees of sweating, warmth and/or coolness, flushing, discoloration, and shiny skin.

    The way that CRPS develops is poorly understood, but theories include irritation and abnormal excitation of the autonomic nervous system, leading to abnormal impulses along nerves. These reduce the diameter of blood vessels that nourish muscles and skin. A variety of events can trigger the condition, including trauma, surgery, heart disease, degenerative arthritis of the neck, and nerve irritation by entrapment (such as carpal tunnel syndrome). CRPS is not rare, and it can imitate sciatica in places where pain is felt and in its distribution on the skin. This condition can also cause a bewildering array of symptoms that don't follow any known pattern.

THE MOST COMMON CAUSE OF SCIATICA

For many years physicians have agreed that the most common origin of sciatica is at the vertebrae in the back—L4, L5, and S1—though this idea is beginning to be challenged.[15] The lumbar spine does most of its job there, supports more weight there, sustains more muscular force exerted just above there, is quite mobile there, and has variable clearance between nerve and bone. In addition, the vertebral disks are bigger there, and because of that they require thicker walls to remain intact. Therefore this is the spot that seems to be the most vulnerable to disk problems that injure the nerves. Although there is no proof that disk changes in this spot (or in others) are absolutely linked with aging, or that disk problems are linked to factors other than growing older, there are indications that diminished blood supply to these areas results in tissue breakdown that begins inside the disk during the second half of a person's life.[16]

REFERRED PAIN

The pain or other discomfort you may be feeling, likely as a result of damage to a spinal disk, that radiates down into your leg or foot is very real and unpleasant. However, it's not necessarily what it seems. What you feel in the lower part of your body may be a manifestation of a problem that is higher up. The cause of the pain is most often in the back—from damage to or compression ("pinching") of those nerve fibers exiting the spinal column—even though you may be feeling the discomfort in another place entirely.

When describing the nature of sciatica, my favorite analogy is to a telephone landline. You may be sitting on the sofa in your living room in New York, talking to someone in San Francisco. But a lineman doing repairs at that moment in Kansas might cause static that disrupts your call. It would be completely understandable for you to say to your friend in California, "What's happening out there? Sounds like an earthquake." After all, how could you know that the cause of the problem was in Kansas? Your connection is to California, and that's the call on which you're hearing the noises.

The same kind of phenomenon occurs in the brain, which locates the signals of pain along the nerve fibers at the spot from which those fibers generally receive signals. If the fibers serve the foot, you will feel the pain in your foot, even though the actual injury is in the spine. This means that a problem in your back that affects the fibers that will form the sciatic nerve may cause you to feel pain in your right thigh and calf, or in your left and right thigh and calf, depending on what region those nerve fibers serve.

Doctors, aware of this fact of biology, are actually able to "work backward" and locate the source of the pain much more accurately than if they simply examined the place where it hurts.

Nerves grow out of each side of the spine at every level, and we are all hardwired. At each level the nerves that depart from the spinal cord are destined for almost exactly the same spot in every person on Earth. Nerve fibers from L5-S1, for example, serve the very outside of the foot and the little toe in everyone. See the diagram on page 63 and look for a more detailed discussion of this later.

If you can say that the brain makes a "mistake" when it interprets something happening in the back as a pain in the foot, the brain makes a similar "mistake" when a heart attack occurs, locating the pain in the shoulder, the left little finger, or the jaw. If you pull your child out of the path of a speeding car and strike your "funny bone" on a parking meter, you feel an electric shock in your ring finger and pinky. That's not because your municipality has wired the sidewalk for sound. You have traumatized the ulnar nerve, overstimulating fibers that normally report signals from your hand. Furthermore, if you strike your elbow hard enough, those fibers will be injured, and it is your pinky that will be numb. The cause is at the elbow, but the manifestation is in the hand. In addition, research shows that a problem on one side of the body can stimulate a trigger point that causes changes on the other side of the body. The cause there too is mediated by the central nervous system and, again, is far from where the pain is felt.[17]

MIMICS OF SCIATICA

Sciatica is not a muscle spasm, a bruise, or a broken bone, although pain from all these problems may produce pain down the leg and masquerade as sciatica. Many other causes of pain along the course of the sciatic nerve have nothing to do with the nerve itself. If you have pain down the leg, into the foot, it may be because of an injury in the back or buttock that is affecting the nerve, and therefore it may be true sciatica. On the other hand, the pain may be due to hamstring sprain or strain, or (rarely) sacroiliac joint derangement or ischial bursitis or, even more rarely, a tumor. It may be hip arthritis or muscle spasm, or anything that affects the posterior femoral cutaneous nerve, which is near the sciatic nerve. In these cases it is you as a "diagnostician," not the brain, that may misidentify the pain as sciatica.

For example, an educated patient came to me recently and said that his knee hurt. He had already seen another doctor and had a diagnostic MRI (magnetic resonance imaging). The MRI showed no problem with his knee. "I think I have sciatica," this gentleman told me. I knew that couldn't be right, because the sciatic nerve doesn't serve the part of the knee that hurt. So, I did further tests and discovered that the man was right about the pain having its origins in his back. Actually he was mistaking the name but not the nature of the pain he was feeling. A herniated disk higher up in his spine was causing the knee pain. That is, pressure on nerve fibers in his spine was causing pain at a distant spot that the injured fibers served. It turned out that fibers of his femoral (not his sciatic) nerve were damaged, and a course of oral steroids and physical therapy provided relief.

Basically, there are four types of problems that mimic but are not sciatic pain.

1. **MUSCULAR PROBLEMS.** Pulled or sprained muscles or a muscle spasm can cause pain that goes from the buttock down the back of the leg, across the knee, and down to the ankle or foot. This type of pain can arise from a particularly vigorous hike.

2. **VASCULAR PROBLEMS.** Problems with the blood vessels can cause pain that seems like sciatica. Claudication, which occurs chiefly in the calf when walking, is a good example. It happens because there isn't enough arterial blood to feed active muscles oxygen and glucose and get rid of the by-products of metabolism. The pain stops when you stop walking. If this is happening to you, you will know because the pain almost always arises with the same amount of walking. If the pain always starts after walking—say two blocks to the grocery store—and it ceases if you stop there and rest, what you've got probably isn't sciatica.

Some people are tempted to have surgery for claudication, but the risk is high for clots, which could lead to amputation down the road. I favor slowly increasing the time and distance that you walk. Walk until it hurts, then stop. Do it twice a day, and you will find that you can double your range within three months.

Another vascular mimic of sciatica happens when an injury causes a Compartment Syndrome. A soccer player who is kicked in the shin might find that the calf swells enough to limit the vascular supply, endangering the muscles and nerves. This is fairly unmistakable because of the swelling, the acute context, and the nature of the pain. It is often treated surgically, and quickly, to decompress the lower leg.

3. **CHRONIC EDEMA (swelling caused by extra fluid).** This can be caused by congestive heart failure or peripheral vascular disease; it can make your legs feel heavy, and make them hurt because they *are* heavy. They weigh more because fluid has collected in them. This of course is not sciatica, but it can produce the same feeling. Ironically, if your legs get heavy enough, lifting them during daily activities, such as walking, can cause back pain.

4. **NEUROPATHIC CONDITIONS.** Weak, uncoordinated, and ineffective transmission of motor and sensory impulses in a single nerve, including the sciatic nerve but also other single nerves, can mimic sciatica.

THE EMOTIONAL COMPONENT

Although there is absolutely no doubt that sciatica is a physiological problem with material causes, there is an emotional factor. General well-being and even job satisfaction have been shown to be related to the severity and duration of back pain.

Two patients who came to my office suffering from extreme back pain and sciatica had an experience in common. One suffered his first injury while serving as a pallbearer at his father's funeral. The other, while helping his dying father shift in his hospital bed, became subject to severe back pain and sciatica, which went on for years. In spite of the knowledge that their back pain had an emotional aspect, these men had real physical discomfort. Knowledge didn't provide a magic cure. Sometimes a patient's back pain has an emotional factor that the person doesn't want to acknowledge. Stress and depression are often manifested in various physical symptoms, including back pain.

The relationship between back pain and the emotions has been the lifework of John Sarno, MD, a professor of clinical rehabilitation medicine at New York University School of Medicine and an attending physician at the Howard A. Rusk Institute of Rehabilitation Medicine. According to Dr. Sarno, emotions influence the amount of pain a person feels and how he or she copes with that pain. Unexpressed anger, especially, or disappointment may prolong or intensify back pain. In cases where muscles are habitually tensed, these emotions may even be responsible for the pain.

A famous research study showed that many individuals have herniated disks but no pain.[18] Often we contract our muscles and compress our nerves, but no spasm or pain results. One explanation for these situations is that the context is not conducive to feeling the unpleasant sensations. While sitting in the library and studying, you might see a beautiful woman entering the room. This could change the way you think of the description in the book you are reading of a man lying down in the desert to feel the "wind blowing over him." When the context—the frame around your perceptions—changes, the perceptions themselves may be transformed. That is part of what John Sarno is saying. I have sent Dr. Sarno many patients, and nearly all of them have benefited significantly. If you have a herniated disk, you may find that you highlight those aspects of your condition that are physically uncomfortable. You might psychologically try to change the context so that the physical discomfort is no longer in the forefront. Another possibility is patiently working to relocate the material that has escaped from the disk or has been displaced, so it is no longer in contact with the nerves. Or you may have the disk removed.

According to Dr. Herbert Benson, the founding president of the Mind/Body Medical Institute, and associate professor of medicine, Harvard Medical School, regular elicitation of the relaxation response has been scientifically proven to be an effective treatment for a wide range of stress-related disorders. In fact, to the extent that any disease is caused or made worse by stress, the relaxation response can help.

Expectations about treatment—another emotional factor—can also influence outcomes. In 1999, an article published in the *Journal of General Internal Medicine*[19] compared expectations of 273 patients who had surgery to relieve sciatica. Patients who expected symptom relief and a short recovery from their operation were twice as likely to be pleased or delighted with their outcomes a year later as patients who had lower expectations. Researchers concluded that although physicians' expectations for surgery were sometimes overly optimistic when weighed against what patients themselves reported about their experience afterward, patients who had a more positive attitude toward surgery to relieve sciatica were more likely to benefit from that surgery.

THE UNCONSCIOUS VERSUS THE SUBCONSCIOUS

There is yet another area where back problems reside, somewhere between repressed anger and other psychological factors, and clear-cut medical causes. Through no fault of his own, and in spite of his prodigious and brilliant work on the human psyche, Sigmund Freud did the medical profession a lasting disservice when he identified the subconscious without distinguishing it from what I'll call the "not conscious." Often we attribute thoughts and feelings to things bubbling up through the subconscious—a mysterious, unknown entity that we alternately believe is our enemy or an expression of what we really are or what we really feel. Although there may be some truth in this—and I think there is—there is also something else.

Many things in our lives slip from consciousness to another level, which has nothing to do with what Freud was talking about when he defined the subconscious. For example, when you learn to drive a car, you consciously shift from one gear to another, you click on the turn signal by actively recalling that you're supposed to do so, and you turn left or right the same way. When you learn to speak a foreign language, at first you have to think carefully about every word and its pronunciation. After a while, as with using the computer keyboard or learning to knit, the action becomes "automatic." The same sort of process happens when you walk, bathe, dress, and eat.

This is also what happens when muscles go into spasm. When you have muscle spasm, there may be unexpressed rage or depression on a subconscious level, but there is also a lack of awareness of the physical contraction. After physical therapy and changes brought about by pain-reducing injections, you can gradually learn to establish some conscious contact, to make the contraction and relaxation of that muscle more voluntary and accessible. You can take your mind off the pain and focus instead on muscle control. Making the state of the muscle conscious is what allows you to learn to control it in the same way you learn to control your bowel movements. You don't think about it all the time. You just do it. You've been taught. This applies in particular to the piriformis muscle. Usually an injection to relax it makes you aware of how that feels, so you can try to reproduce the feeling. Physical therapy may also help establish contact—a conscious awareness of the muscle—again. Surgery removes the muscle so no control is necessary.

SCIATICA MIXTURES AND MIMICS

Some conditions are a mix of nerve pain and other problems. It's possible to have sciatica or pain associated with other nerves, and at the same time to have something else. For example, suppose you have pain in your legs that occurs when you're walking and resolves when you stop walking. That might be a condition called claudication, which I've discussed as a mimic of sciatica and is related to poor blood circulation in the arteries in the leg. Leg pain that can be confused with sciatica can be caused by vascular disease, as well as by nerve compression in your spine. But sometimes it's not that simple.

By the time the sciatic nerve reaches the back of the knee, it has divided in two. One branch travels down the leg right next to the top of the fibular bone, which is known as the fibular head. This is a frequent site of entrapment. Compression can occur when people cross their legs, or when they have fallen backward. If that is the situation, the patient has two complaints: funny feelings, tingling, burning, unpleasant sensations of stiffness in the side of the leg, or difficulty lifting the foot when taking a step forward. Are the strange sensations or muscle weakness sciatica or not? Well, they are due to injury of the sciatic nerve, but have a separate, local explanation.

Although these people have sensory symptoms that are closely associated with sciatica, and motor symptoms that go along with it as well, an MRI might be mystifyingly normal. An expert assessing this situation is likely to say that the funny feelings on the outside of the leg come from L5-S1, but the inability to lift the foot comes from L4-L5. Maybe some experts are reluctant to call it sciatica because those are two different levels of the spine. They might both be involved, but it is more common in medicine, as everywhere else, to find a single cause for multiple phenomena. In this case those fibers, L4-L5, go to the anterior tibialis muscle, which lifts the foot, and the L5-S1 fibers that serve the outside of the calf travel together in the peroneal nerve and are frequently entrapped at the little bone—the fibular head.

THE RELATIONSHIP BETWEEN SCIATICA AND BACK PAIN

Although there is a tremendous difference between sciatica and back pain, there is also a lot of overlap. Back pain is in the back; sciatica is pain along the course of the sciatic nerve in the buttock and down the leg. So, geographically you can place them in different parts of the body. They're distinct. But these two symptoms frequently occur together and frequently have a common cause. In other words, a herniated disk in your back can give you a backache and sciatica. The cause of the pain is in your back, and your back hurts right there. When the pain goes down your leg, you've got sciatica.

Chapter III

THE NERVOUS SYSTEM AND SELF-DIAGNOSIS

FIRST, HERE IS A SHORT lesson in the anatomical components of the nervous system. If you have sciatica, it's likely that your physician will use one or more of these words or phrases. They can be confusing; it's good to have some understanding of them, so when you hear them in your doctor's office, you have an idea of what they mean.

BASIC COMPONENTS OF THE NERVOUS SYSTEM

NEURON: A nerve cell—the building block of the nervous system. It consists of a cell body, containing the nucleus, all the DNA, and at least two long processes, or filaments—dendrites, which carry signals toward the cell body, and axons, which carry signals away.

CENTRAL NERVOUS SYSTEM: The neurons contained in the brain and spinal cord.

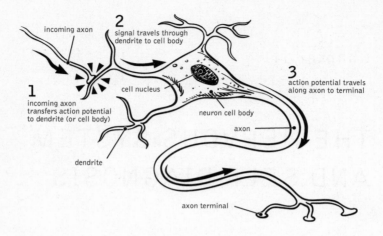

All neurons are the same; they are stimulated at the dendrites (1) and transmit signals through the cell body (2) to the end of the axon (3).

PERIPHERAL NEURONS: All other neurons not in the brain or spinal cord.

MOTOR NEURONS: Nerve cells that carry signals from the central nervous system to muscles and glands.

SENSORY NEURONS: These nerve cells carry signals from the eyes, ears, mucous membranes, skin, joints, muscles, and internal organs toward the cell body, and then from the cell body onward toward the central nervous system.

SCIATIC NERVE: Consists of sensory and motor neurons that carry motor signals from the brain through the back to the muscles of the legs, and sensory signals upward from the leg, through the spinal cord, to the brain.

Fibers that normally send signals to the brain from their specially adapted nerve endings in the skin of the calf are stimulated by the herniated disk as they enter the bony spine between L4 and L5. The brain interprets the signals caused by the disk's pressure on the nerves as coming from the calf, even though the cause of the pain is in the spine.

nerve root compression

sciatic nerve

peroneal division

tibial division

referred pain

NERVE ROOTLETS: In the lumbar spine, the nerve fibers that travel to the legs do so in small bundles. Each little bundle is called a nerve rootlet, and the whole accumulation of bundles was thought by some fanciful anatomist to resemble the tail of a horse, so this collection throughout the lumbar spine is called the "cauda equina." In a diagnostic MRI, you can see these little bundles of nerve fibers.

NERVE ROOTS: Bundles of nerve rootlets fuse together when leaving the spine through one of the small openings between vertebrae called the neuroforamina. At this point these collections of nerve rootlets, composed of motor and sensory cells about as thick as a pencil, are termed nerve roots.

LUMBOSACRAL PLEXUS: Where the nerve roots join with one another in the space behind the sacroiliac joints, and the nerve fibers within them redistribute themselves into the collections that form the sciatic nerve and other nerves of the pelvis and lower extremities.

Researchers agree that sciatica is neurological in origin. To exist, it needs the brain, the spinal cord, the peripheral nerves in the legs, and the pathways that connect them to one another.

The brain and spinal cord make up the central nervous system (CNS). In babies the spinal cord extends to the bottom of the bony spinal canal, L5-S1. But the bones grow more than the nerves do, and the spinal cord itself ends up at the level of T12. (See illustration on page 28.) From there on down, the peripheral fibers are stretched into the long strands of rootlets—the cauda equina. These fibers are inside the bony canal at the level of the lumbar spine, but they are not really in the central nervous system.

The nerve fibers leaving the central nervous system travel down through the lumbar spine and, as roots, enter the lumbosacral plexus. When they exit this anatomical hub, the fibers have regrouped into the peripheral nerves. All the nerves that aren't in the brain or spine— the sciatic nerve, the femoral nerve, and all other nerve components in the arms and legs—are in the peripheral nervous system.

The central nervous system is where most of the nerve cells, or neurons, are located. These neurons work hard, receiving, organizing, grouping, critically evaluating, remembering, and—on occasion—making things up. They have helper cells that nourish them, and linings and bony coverings that insulate them from the chemical and physical changes of the rest of the body, and they are bathed in special fluids with their own circulation.

These neurons take in information from outside and inside the body, then determine what to do with it—in conscious and unconscious ways. Neurons also have the tricky job of designating what comes up to consciousness, and what does not. The nonconscious activities, including digestion and blood flow, are of course neurologically controlled; the part of the system responsible for that control used to be rather rigidly designated the autonomic nervous system. However, now, because of the awareness of the psychological aspect of many types of pain, this distinction is more flexible.

Neurons are the building blocks of the nervous system; they are so valuable to us that nature has provided them with ample protection. After the neurons' long, tendril-like processes have emerged from the protective bony covering of the spinal cord at the lumbosacral plexus, Schwann cells—soft insulating cells—wrap themselves around the neurons. The Schwann cells also speed the neurons' signals.

All motor nerve cell bodies are located in the central nervous system —the spinal cord and brain. Usually there is a chain of two or three neurons between the brain and the muscle that wiggles the toe (and many modulating connections along the way), but all of the motor nerve cells are within the bony coverings. The last link in the chain sends out a long tendril that stimulates the muscle to act. For instance, the tendril

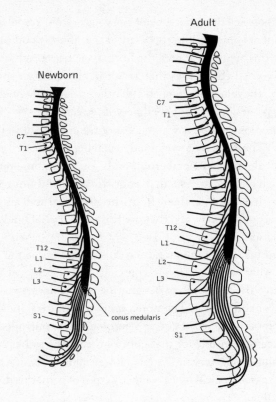

The spinal cord itself grows less than the bones that protect it.
The dendrites of the sensory fibers and the axons of the motor
fibers extend as the vertebrae grow.

between vertebrae L5 and S1, which extends all the way down to the
flexor muscles of the calf, can make those muscles move.

Weakness and other problems traceable to muscles are an important
"insult added to injury" when it comes to sciatica. Footdrop, which
shows up clearly when the patient is walking or climbing stairs, is
common.

The central nervous system's neurons—both motor and sensory—
extend only from the brain to the end of the thoracic spine, near the
level of the twelfth rib. Little bundles of nerve fibers travel from those

cells through the lumbar spinal canal, then out to the muscles and skin of the legs. These little bundles, called rootlets, are the only neurological inhabitants of the lumbar spine. As these bundles of nerve fibers leave the safe confines of the spine, they are grouped together into soft cables about as big around as a pencil, and become "nerve roots." These roots exit the spine symmetrically between each two vertebrae, more or less resembling a Christmas tree in their balanced branching (see illustration below).

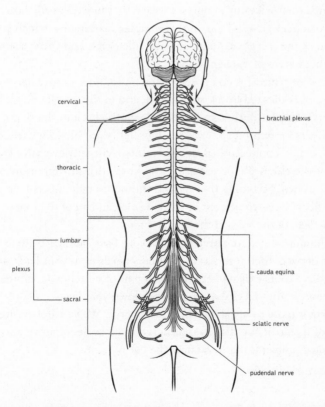

Fibers descend from the level of their roots in the spine and reorganize in the lumbosacral plexus. Fibers from each level are destined to enter exactly the same nerve and serve exactly the same muscles, skin, and bones in every person.

Something unusual happens once the nerve fibers leave the spine on their way to the lumbosacral plexus. The cell bodies of the sensory nerves join the motor fibers, extending some fibers (dendrites) out to the leg, and other fibers (axons) the other way, back to the spinal cord on their way to the brain. So the motor and sensory fibers travel together, but they originate in different locations. And they connect separately to different parts of the brain.

Once the motor and sensory fibers of the different lumbar roots on each side of the lumbosacral plexus join with one another, they rearrange themselves in a complex weave that resembles the on-and-off ramps of a freeway. It is here, in this complex rearranging, which goes on in front of the sacroiliac joints on each side of the body, that the sciatic and other nerves of the legs form.

The sciatic nerve is composed of the motor and sensory nerve fibers whose cell bodies are in the spinal cord, and in the ganglia beside it. As the nerve extends farther and farther down the back of the thigh, some of its fibers branch off to serve the muscles, skin, blood vessels, sweat glands, bones, connective tissue, and joints—virtually everything in the back of the thigh. Before crossing the knee, this all-important nerve divides in two, becoming thinner and thinner as more fibers branch off. These fibers serve 75 percent of the lower leg and all of the foot muscles and the skin of the soles of the feet and toes.

To sum up, there are nerve fibers in your back, and then there is the sciatic nerve, which forms as those fibers reach from your back to your legs. Nerve roots exiting between each pair of vertebrae combine with the fibers of other roots that then travel down your legs.

There is more to say about the sciatic nerve. We've barely visited the place of its birth! We discuss that nerve in more detail as we cover the individual problems that can affect the back.

HOW TO FIGURE OUT IF YOU
HAVE SCIATICA

You can see your doctor. You can have diagnostic tests. But you can also do a lot yourself to find out if you have sciatica. Once you have the answer, you can look for a cure. Frequently a single factor may make the case for sciatica. Often, however, you and your physician need all the information you can get to lead you toward a diagnosis.

Merriam-Webster's Collegiate Dictionary defines sciatica as "pain in the region of the hips or along the course of the nerve at the back of the thigh." To most physicians, and therefore to the patients who wish to communicate with them, sciatica is pain and related discomforts due to some abnormality affecting the sciatic nerve or its constituents. Remember, we are speaking of a particular nerve. To figure out whether you have sciatica, consider the following.

* Pain or discomfort along the path of the sciatic nerve and any of its way stations, including the muscles and skin it serves. See illustration on page 25.
* Numbness: Loss of feeling. Sometimes this can be subtle. Often my patients are surprised to discover they have areas of numbness on their legs or feet. You can test for this yourself with the edge of a matchbook or a toothpick, comparing areas of skin on one leg with the same areas on the other leg.
* Parasthesias: Strange sensations, including electric-shock-like feelings, tingling, pins and needles, burning, "bugs crawling," and "pinching."
* Weakness: Unusual lack of strength that may cause your knees to buckle when you're standing up or may make it difficult to rise from a sitting position. Inability to walk on heels or toes. You may find that when walking your feet don't have their normal strength.
* Reduced reflexes: Your doctor most often tests reflexes—the Achilles tendon reflex (sciatic nerve L5-S1) can be compared with the other side and with the knee reflex (femoral nerve L2, L3, L4)—but you can do these at home with at least some degree of accuracy.

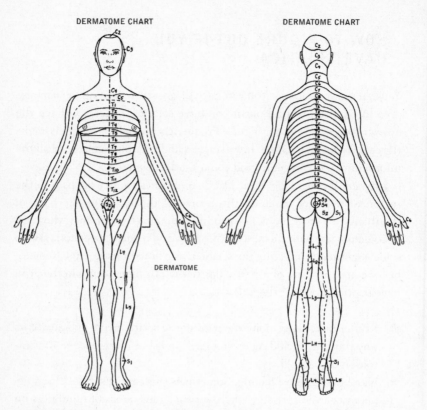

DERMATOME CHART   DERMATOME CHART

DERMATOME

Specific nerve roots from different spinal levels serve separate parts of the foot and leg, and specific nerves carry the nerve fibers. Numbness and tingling usually follow these outlines, and give a big hint about which spinal level or which nerve has the injury responsible for your pain.

The Achilles tendon reflex is elicited by striking the Achilles tendon with a soft mallet and observing the ankle flexion that results. The patellar reflex swings the shin up of a sitting person after the tendon is struck just below the kneecap.

* Fatigue in your leg: Also feeling that your leg is no longer part of you. "It's like it's somebody else's leg."

* Footdrop: Can't walk on your heels, or (less commonly), your toes.

COMMON PATTERNS OF SCIATICA
AND THEIR CAUSES

1. Pain and pins and needles down the outside of the calf to the first toe web space; poor heel or toe walking. (Spinal problems or piriformis syndrome.)
2. Burning in back of thigh and calf to heel with stiff legs. Possible difficulty walking on toes. (Spinal problems or piriformis syndrome.)
3. Pain sitting with tingling at the back of the thigh, relieved by standing, with numbness in all the toes. (Piriformis syndrome.)
4. Buttock and sciatic pain with running, gym/health club working out, and/or protracted driving. No numbness, weakness, or tingling. (Piriformis syndrome.)
5. Pain in mid–lower back with painful electric shocks down part or all of the course of the sciatic nerve, possibly with tingling, burning, weakness, and numbness. (Acute herniated disk.)
6. Pain or burning at the outside of the lower thighs and sides of the calf, with stiff back. (Spinal stenosis.)

On page 34 is a diagnosis diagram, typical of what is used in medical school to teach doctors how to find the cause of a certain symptom or symptoms. As with a decision tree, you make a decision (usually yes or no) at each branch. Here we're trying to figure out what causes sciatica. For example, the first question is, does the symptom go below the knee? If the answer is no, the pain probably (and I must emphasize the word "probably" with all these decisions) isn't from piriformis syndrome or any neurological cause. If the answer is yes, that the pain does go below the knee, you should look at the upper middle portion of the diagram and ask yourself if there's a tender buttock, weak abduction (bringing leg out from the midline), and painful adduction (weakness when pulling the leg in) of the thigh. If the answer is yes, you probably have piriformis syndrome.

Look at the bottom of the diagram. There is a list of decisions to make after understanding that nerve roots actually are pinched. The L1, L2,

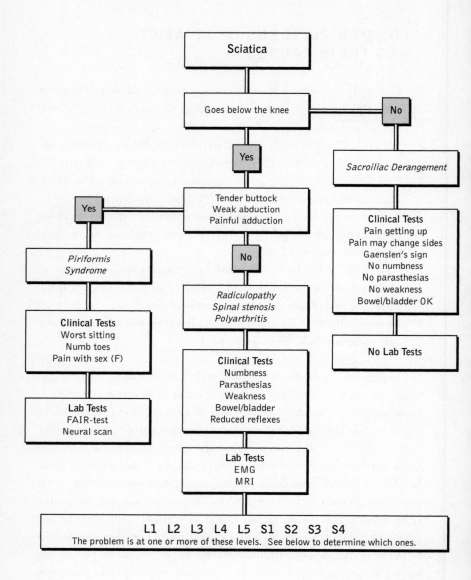

This is a diagnosis diagram for sciatica, listing its major causes.
Musculoskeletal pain does not cause sciatica.

WEAKNESS:

Flexing the thigh: DIAGNOSIS—RADICULOPATHY AT L1-L2

Extending the knee: DIAGNOSIS—RADICULOPATHY AT L2, 3, 4

Raising the foot at the ankle: DIAGNOSIS—RADICULOPATHY AT L4-L5

Walking on the toes: DIAGNOSIS—RADICULOPATHY AT L5-S1

Difficulty controlling the bowel or bladder: DIAGNOSIS—S1, 2, 3

PRESCRIPTION: EACH CONDITION MAY BE TREATED WITH MCKENZIE EXERCISES APPROPRIATE FOR THE LEVEL AND SEVERITY OF INJURY. BUT SUDDEN LOSS OF BOWEL, BLADDER, OR LIMB CONTROL IS A SURGICAL EMERGENCY.

NUMBNESS AND/OR PARASTHESIAS:

Inguinal region, including side of testicle, labia majoris: L1

Upper front and side of thigh: L2

Main region of front of thigh down to and/or including knee: L3

Inside of calf, top of foot: L4-L5

First web space, very outside of foot, outside of calf: S1

Middle back of thigh: S2

Middle portion of testicles, penis, anus: S3

Head of penis, clitoris: S4

THE FOLLOWING INDICATE PIRIFORMIS SYNDROME:

Weakness, numbness, or parasthesias from L4-S2

Pain worse sitting than standing

Pace's sign means weak abduction. This happens when a person has piriformis syndrome. When it's more difficult to bring one leg up from the bed (that is, that leg is weaker), there is piriformis syndrome on that side. When trying to diagnose piriformis syndrome on both sides, muscle strength has to be looked at in proportion to other muscles. (See page 75.)

Solheim's sign: Pain in the buttock with passive adduction and internal rotation of the flexed thigh. Evidence favoring piriformis syndrome.

Numbness and/or parasthesias in the toes, rather than the feet, often suggests piriformis syndrome rather than nerve root compression at the spinal cord.[20]

Even though piriformis syndrome and other conditions can coexist, a negative MRI and a negative standard EMG strongly suggest a diagnosis of piriformis syndrome as a cause of sciatica. A recent study found that 67 percent of nonspinal sciatica was due to piriformis syndrome.[21]

THE FOLLOWING SUGGEST A DIAGNOSIS OF SPINAL STENOSIS:

Pain that is bilateral and by and large symmetrical.

Weakness, numbness, and parasthesias indicate multiple levels of involvement, some on each side.

Pain that is worse when the person is stretched out (either standing or lying down) rather than bent, as in sitting.

The MRI and EMG go a long way in helping to sort out the diagnosis when multiple symptoms appear.

ARTHRITIS MAY ALSO CAUSE A MULTILEVEL RADICULOPATHY OR PINCHED NERVE ROOTS:

Imaging studies are the only way to tell for sure.

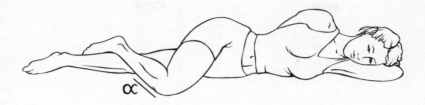

Flexion, adduction, and internal rotation stretch the piriformis muscle tight, compressing the sciatic nerve. The solid angle alpha α is directly proportional to the force of this compression.

and so on at the bottom of the diagram requires a further explanation. You need to identify the level of the injury. That's what the box on pages 35–36 is all about.

The box shows each level, starting with L1 and going to S4, and lists symptoms and signs, muscle strength (motor nerves), feelings (sensory nerves), reflexes, et cetera. By looking at the box, you can tell the level of the injury, having been guided to the answer from the decisions you made throughout the diagram. This information is supplemented and described again in the chart on motor root levels (see page 63). Look for more explanation following the chart.

Chapter IV

DIAGNOSTIC TESTS
AND NERVE FUNCTION

WHAT SHOULD YOU DO IF YOU THINK YOU HAVE SCIATICA?

The first thing to do if you think you have sciatica is to look for the cause of this symptom. The more you know about what is making you feel that tingling, numbness, weakness, burning, or other discomfort, the greater the possibility of getting relief. Go to your doctor, and make sure that he or she takes a complete medical history, including information about any past episodes of back pain or sciatica, tingling, numbness, and weakness.

A full physical examination should be done. During this exam, your doctor will attempt to rule out some potentially serious medical conditions, such as tumor, infection, and fracture. He or she may want to observe you as you sit and as you walk in order to evaluate your posture and gait. The range of motion in your back should be checked. And your spine, buttock, and leg may be touched in various places, looking for tenderness and spasm.

There are several major ways that doctors attempt to characterize sciatica during a physical exam. Pain or discomfort over the "sciatic notch," the place where the sciatic nerve begins (see illustration of L-S-plexus on page 29), may indicate some irritation of the nerve itself or its roots.

Sciatica begins near the spot where the sciatic nerve exits the pelvis, between the sacrum and the iliac bones. The sciatic nerve moves downward from there and usually ducks underneath the piriformis muscle on its way out of the pelvis and toward the back of the leg, although about 15 percent of the time the nerve actually goes through the muscle. Most people who have piriformis syndrome have pain and tenderness there, where muscle and nerve intersect.

You may be asked by your doctor to walk on your heels, then on your toes, in a test of muscle strength and possible nerve dysfunction. Ankle jerk reflex and knee jerk reflex tests may also be performed to check for possible nerve problems.

The classic "straight leg raise test" may also be administered. You are asked to lie on your back on the examining table. One by one, the physician will raise your legs, watching to see if pain occurs and, if it does, at what angle and where. If the angle is between 30 and 60 degrees and the pain is in the back, it often indicates irritation of nerve roots that form the sciatic nerve. Bending the knee while the leg is still raised should relieve the pain. If it does not relieve the pain, the problem is probably in the hip. If the pain is in the back of your knee and occurs at the same angle for both legs, you may have nothing more serious than tight hamstrings.

Based on the results of the straight leg test, your doctor may be able to say that you are suffering from sciatica from certain probable causes, although more diagnostic tests may need to be done to identify the exact location and nature of the injury to the nerve's fibers.

Here I must say that although internists—extremely sophisticated diagnosticians who can identify obscure types of hepatitis and thyroid or kidney abnormalities—are often able to spot sciatica, that is not their specialty. They often prescribe a nonsteroidal anti-inflammatory and a medication to relax muscles, and those approaches often work. If they don't work, I recommend an appointment with a specialist in physical medicine and rehabilitation or with a neurologist. If you believe that you have sciatica, and the pain and discomfort haven't gone away after 2 weeks, many internists will consent to send you to a specialist.

Some problems necessitate surgery. If you have sciatica and begin to experience other symptoms, such as difficulty walking, increasingly numb or weak legs, or problems with bowel or urinary control, you may have the rare cauda equina syndrome, which is a surgical emergency, although this is not likely. A recent five-year Danish study found that it occurred in only one in 1.3 million people in Denmark.[22] If you have a severely herniated disk and unremitting pain, you may need to see a surgeon. Read more about surgery in Chapter X.

DIAGNOSTIC TESTS

There are several common diagnostic tests that are done to find out what is causing sciatica. The EMG (electromyography) and MRI are the most common exams used for identifying nerve injury, though in some cases an X-ray, a bone scan, or a CT (computerized tomography) scan may also be valuable, and the newer "neuroimaging" is available to examine the pelvis more accurately. Although the EMG is an excellent diagnostic test that can reveal the causes of sciatica, it doesn't show the problem immediately. If you had an EMG the day you came down with severe back pain, for example, it could show some types of injury but not others. If you have back pain and are considering an EMG, you should wait 2 to 3 weeks before having the test, to give a complete picture.

EMG: WHAT IT IS

EMG, or electromyography, literally means in Greek "electric picture of a muscle." There are two parts to this test. The first part measures how fast and how completely nerves conduct their impulses. It shows whether or not muscles are receiving all the impulses being sent to them and also whether the sensory nerves are doing their job. It shows whether there is a weakened or slowed impulse and, if so, where the weakening or slowing occurs. It also determines whether there is a full signal and/or whether any signal at all is getting through.

The second part of the EMG uses a tiny Teflon-coated antenna that is inserted into the muscles themselves to see whether they are giving off characteristic signals that indicate nerve damage. This part of the test reveals whether any nerve fibers have been cut or are significantly damaged by picking up and amplifying signals that originate in the muscles. This is discussed further below.

Once I did an EMG on an electrician. When I gave him the initial stimulus, I turned to him and asked, "Is that all right?" "Yes," he replied. "But, Doc, could you turn up the juice a little?" That man was in the right profession. Another time, when one of my sons was nine, I had a new EMG device delivered to my home. My son was fascinated, and kept cajoling me to tell him about it, then to show him how it worked, and finally to let him see what it felt like. Naturally I resisted; he persisted. Finally I gave in and attached an electrode to the muscle in his calf, and let him feel the stimulation. I felt like the worst father in the world, but he seemed to like it.

In general, almost all patients young and old are able to tolerate the small electric stimuli that come with having an EMG. Occasionally someone, especially someone overworked and exhausted, becomes relaxed enough to fall asleep during the test.

EMG: WHAT IT SHOWS

All of us humans are hard wired, all built the same way, with few variations. In almost every individual, a given muscle is commanded to contract by nerve fibers that come from the same vertebral level. The medical profession has learned the anatomical diagram. So, from the data acquired through doing an EMG with a few muscles, and by examining the conduction characteristics for a small number of nerves, a physician can form an exact picture of what's wrong and how serious it is.

A typical conclusion on an EMG report may be, "Damage at the nerve root between the 4th and 5th lumbar vertebrae on the left," or "Normal study suggesting musculoskeletal causes [for pain]." These conclusions are logically deduced from the responses detected by the EMG instrument.

The first part of the two-part EMG is based on the work of Sir Charles Sherrington, who won the Nobel Prize in 1922 for his work on the giant squid axon. Applying brief electrical impulses to a squid's 12-foot-long single nerve fiber (axon), visible to the naked eye, Sherrington observed twitches in a small muscle fiber on the other end of the axon. He correctly concluded that nerves conduct impulses in much the same fashion that copper wires conduct electricity. He was not far from right, and that concept led to the initial part of the EMG test, in which nerve conduction is timed and the impulse intensity is estimated.

In an EMG, nerves along the arms or legs are stimulated, and the speed and size of the impulses they conduct are measured. Using simple arithmetic (distance = rate × time), it's easy to figure out the rate of conduction along nerve fibers.

If an impulse in one nerve is slow, or small, the question becomes: what about the other nerves? If the impulses of many are slow, there is a problem with the nerves themselves. This is called a neuropathy. If only one or two nerves conduct slowly, and the slowing occurs only at one particular section of the nerve, that's a different kettle of fish. In that case, probably something local is compressing the nerve—for example, an entrapment such as carpal tunnel syndrome. If the speed of conduction is diminished throughout the nerve, it's another type of problem, such as a diabetic neuropathy (mononeuropathy monoplex) or Guillain-Barré syndrome.

But what if the nerve root is compressed as it exits the spine? The nerve fibers in the leg will still function normally. However, if the nerve damage has severed any of the motor nerve fibers, the portion of the fiber beyond the break will die, and within a few days will cease to conduct impulses. So the size of the response to stimulation in the muscle will be reduced.

Because of the way they're configured, sensory fibers in the legs will not die from injury to their axons in the spine. These fibers originate outside the spine, in ganglia. However, if serious injury to nerve fibers occurs in the piriformis region, motor and sensory signals will be diminished.

But what about milder, although still very painful, injury that doesn't destroy neurons but is in the spine above the level at which nerves are stimulated?

Noted German neurologist Johann Hoffmann discovered that it is easy to replicate the Achilles tendon reflex with a small electrical stimulus behind the knee. (See illustration on page 45.) In his honor, the reflex is known as the H-reflex. It involves a sensory nerve's conduction all the way up the leg, then within the spinal column to the level of the twelfth rib (a single synapse there with a motor nerve cell), and a return trip by the motor neuron down the spine and leg to the soleus muscle, which flexes the ankle when stimulated. So with a single stimulus, a physician can investigate certain aspects of the leg and the entire lumbar spine. Possibly best of all, the conduction can be compared with the same process on the other leg—an ideal control.

The H-reflex test is diagnostic for pressure on a nerve root in the spine, or for piriformis syndrome, which involves the sciatic nerve in the buttock. Differences between the H-reflex of the right leg and the left leg usually indicate a compression of the L5 nerve root on the slower side. Values are well-tested for bilateral conditions. The H-reflex can be observed to change when the body is in different positions. This is the way piriformis syndrome is diagnosed. First the regular H-reflex is elicited by the physician when the patient is lying facedown; this becomes the control. If stretching the piriformis muscle over the sciatic nerve prolongs the H-reflex of the right leg but not those of the left leg, then there is piriformis syndrome on the right. Values for this maneuver are well-tested for bilateral conditions as well. These tests allow the physician to measure the response in hundred thousandths of a second and millionths of a volt. The results of this sort of test can be replicated. They appear consistently in multiple exams on different days.

The H-reflex can also be observed to change when the body is in different positions. This is the way piriformis syndrome is diagnosed. First the regular H-reflex is elicited by the physician when the patient is lying prone; this becomes the control.

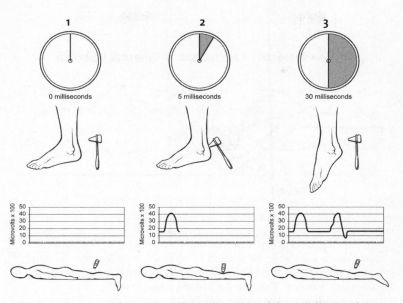

The H-reflex is an electrophysiological version of the Achilles tendon reflex. A small electrical charge (1) stimulates the same fibers that a reflex hammer activates, beginning a reflex (2) that ends with muscle contraction (3), enabling physicians to time the response in hundred thousandths of a second, and measure it in millionths of a volt.

After recording the H-reflex and the time it takes for the reflex to be completed, the patient is placed in flexion, adduction, and internal rotation (the FAIR-test), and the reflex is tested again. For people who do not have sciatica or piriformis syndrome, stretching the piriformis muscle does nothing. The H-reflex remains unchanged. For people who do have this problem, the stretched muscle presses into the sciatic nerve with sufficient force to slow down the H-reflex impulses quite a bit, and the diagnosis for piriformis syndrome can be made relatively easily. See Chapter V for a more complete discussion.

But suppose all the conductions of motor and sensory nerves are normal. The second part of the EMG test is the needle test. This procedure owes its origin to the discovery that when muscles have lost their nervous connection to the spinal cord because of illness or injury, they give

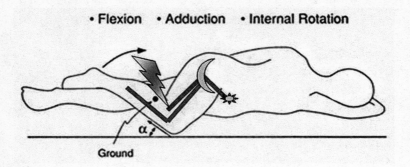

• Flexion   • Adduction   • Internal Rotation

Ground

Stretching the piriformis muscle tightly against the sciatic nerve may compress the nerve enough to delay the H-reflex's sensory limb, going up to the spinal cord, and delay its descending motor limb by the same amount. This will double the effect that the piriformis muscle's pressure has on the H-reflex.

off characteristic signals that are recognized by other, intact nerve fibers, and can be detected on the oscilloscope of the EMG instrument. Because all humans are hard wired, and the same muscles are supplied by the same nerves and the same nerve roots from the same levels of the spine in every one of us, an electromyographer can test various muscles and, from the pattern of missing nerve connections, determine exactly where the injury to the spine (or peripheral nerve) must be.

SSEP

What an EMG does for muscles, the somatosensory evoked potential (SSEP) test does for sensory nerves. These are the nerves that make us aware of feelings of pleasure and pain, and tingling and other unpleasant sensations. As you know, motor signals go from the brain down to the muscles when you want to wiggle your toe or say hello. Sensory signals go the other way, starting in the skin, muscles, joints, or viscera and going upward through the spinal cord to the brain. The SSEP utilizes this, focusing on a specific region of the brain—the somatosensory strip—that receives these signals. This strip is a band that goes side to side across the top of the brain, virtually from one ear to the other, and is organized so that any given point on the body registers at a specific point in the brain. Damage to that part of the brain—for example, from a stroke or a head injury—will show up in an SSEP when electrodes are placed on the scalp. The SSEP is an effective way to detect an injury in the spinal cord that affects only sensory nerves.

Once, during my residency at Albert Einstein Hospital, I had a patient who said she couldn't feel her left arm. Although this brave and lovely woman with three small children had been in a serious automobile accident, she showed few outward signs of emotional upset or physical injury. An EMG had determined conclusively that all her motor fibers were functioning well. She had been having a difficult time with her other doctors and her insurance company, and there had been whispers that she was trying to get sympathy or cash.

Then we did an SSEP, and the results revealed a different story. They showed that the sensory signals were getting through perfectly, until they reached a specific level in her spinal cord, where the sensory fibers had been severed by the wrenching of her neck in one direction and her torso in the other direction. Although these findings got her plenty of sympathy and a good bit of cash, the feeling in her arm never returned. But she had the satisfaction of objective proof that she wasn't crazy or a fraud.

To do an SSEP to test for the cause of sciatica, tiny electrodes—so tiny that three or four of them would fit inside the needle used to give a flu shot—are inserted (almost painlessly) under your skin. Several of these little electrodes are placed above key nerve centers, such as your neck and the base of the spine, along the path leading from your arms and legs back to the somatosensory strip in the brain. Tiny electrodes are also placed on the scalp over the somatosensory strip itself, the last part of the chain of neurons in the brain that actually registers sensations. The somatosensory strip is roughly where a band connecting earphones goes over your head and where sensory input is received by the cerebral cortex. These SSEP electrodes pick up the actual electrical current of nerve impulses when the nerves near your ankles are activated by mild shocks. The electrodes time the impulses' arrival at various points along the nerve path to your brain, and they can also measure the strength of these impulses.

The time it takes for nerve impulses to arrive at various points outside the central nervous system is somewhat variable. However, once the nerves' signals enter the spine, the timing of the impulses is relatively constant in all healthy humans. Delays at any specific spinal level indicate a problem. A delay could be caused by a herniated disk or another injury that interferes with conduction, so that the interval between the arrival of the impulses at one level and another will be lengthened. Delays are easy for doctors to see, and provide much information about where your problem is and how serious it is. By the same token, this test shows where the problem is *not*, which is also valuable information for your doctor.

In other words, if an MRI has already shown that you have a herniated disk between the third and fourth lumbar vertebrae, and that the disk material seems to be pressing against nerve rootlets there, the SSEP can further identify the specific rootlets that are involved. For example, it might tell you that the injured disk is actually pressing on the rootlets that exit farther down on the left side with the L5-S1 nerve root, and it might also indicate that the disk is not really causing the pain at all.

NERVE DAMAGE AND NERVE REGROWTH

How do you and your doctor know whether steroids or physical therapy or just the passage of time are helping your nerves to regenerate? Usually, when individuals have sciatica, they experience good and bad days. The EMG and SSEP are valuable tools for determining what's really happening inside. Repeating the positive parts of these tests periodically to compare nerve conduction timing and impulse size can tell your doctor whether or not you are making progress.

There are three types of nerve damage that can be identified with an

EMG or an SSEP, and the nerves have different possibilities for regrowth and recovery. Sometimes the nerve is just compressed or stretched and temporarily put out of commission, and in time it repairs itself and conducts impulses normally again. There is a name for this situation; it's called neuropraxia. If neuropraxia is present, stimulating the nerve won't get the muscle to react perfectly, or send a full volley of sensory signals toward the brain at normal speed. But the nerve fiber is still alive. When the needle part of the EMG exam is done on that muscle, the muscle will appear to behave normally even though not all impulses are getting through in a timely fashion. A patient with this kind of damage—neuropraxia—can usually expect a complete recovery without treatment in one week to three months.

The second kind of damage occurs when the nerve itself is severed inside its protective, fatty sheath, but the sheath itself remains intact. This breakage or division is caused by tension, pressure, or sometimes other factors, such as oxygen deprivation. Obviously, a broken nerve, even if its sheath is unbroken, will not conduct an impulse when stimulated. There will be signs of Wallerian degeneration inside the sheath. Wallerian is the name for the withering away of nerve tissue that has been cut and severed from the central nervous system. Even though its blood supply is intact, and all other factors are equal, the part(s) of the nerve fibers farther from the spinal cord than the cut will die (and be reabsorbed by the body). As this happens, nerve conduction along that pathway ceases, of course.

But if the sheath that surrounds the nerve fiber is still intact, the nerve fiber will eventually regenerate. In this case, unlike the first case, you will see signs on the EMG of this regrowth as time goes on. Characteristic signals of axonotmesis—the severing of the little nerve fiber in the middle of the sheath—appear on the EMG. The usual regrowth of nerves in a situation like this is about a millimeter a day, or about an inch a month. So if a nerve is cut, say at the piriformis muscle in the buttock, it will have to grow about 1 1/2 to 2 1/2 feet to reach the pre-injury point in the muscles of the calf or foot with which it was previously associated, and to which its sheath leads. That may take 1 1/2 to 2 1/2 years.

The third, more serious type of damage is where the sheath surrounding the fiber and the fiber itself have been severed—cut in two. When this happens, of course there is no conduction of impulses along the nerve, and there will be signs on the EMG that the nerve is not attached to the muscle. There will be Wallerian degeneration of nerve and sheath beyond the point of severance. In this case regrowth is problematical.

When a fall or other kind of accident, or even repetitive running, causes a problem, there may be a combination of all three types of damage. Some nerve fibers will recover on their own, others will regenerate at the rate of an inch a month, and some will not regenerate. But nature is resourceful. Muscle fibers that have no nerve connected to them give off characteristic signals that can show up on an EMG. The muscle also gives off chemical signals to the intact nerves that pass by it—those nerves that escaped damage. These other nerve fibers will respond to the signals and send off little tendrils to the muscle that no longer has a nerve, until another new fiber has grown in place of the one that was destroyed. The new fiber will serve the muscle. These fibers also grow at about a millimeter a day, or an inch a month. That regeneration shows up on an EMG as well.

When the muscle with the regrown nerve tendrils contracts, the muscle is no longer exactly the way it was before the injury. The new tendrils conduct nerve impulses a little more slowly. The muscle will be strong but will likely not regain its complete original physical strength, because all its fibers will not contract simultaneously—unless the patient works on this specifically through exercise in physical therapy. Measuring regeneration of injured nerve fibers with an EMG helps predict future recovery.

MRI: MAGNETIC RESONANCE IMAGING

This painless, safe radiological test uses very strong magnetic fields and ultrasound to make a picture of soft tissue, showing all its outlines and densities in relatively good detail. The picture produced by the MRI machine looks more or less like an X-ray, but with a difference. X-rays pass straight through soft tissue and outline the bones. In MRI, muscles, sinews, blood vessels, and nerves are also visible. You can see with an MRI whether an intervertebral disk, a ligament, or something else is compressing a nerve in a way that may cause a problem. You can also see if swollen tissue is pressing on nearby nerves.

Of course back pain in general and sciatica in particular can be mysterious, and having a trained radiologist and your physician look at your MRI won't necessarily answer all your questions, or theirs. It may not be possible to tell from looking at the picture of the nerve itself whether it is injured. There is a famous study that confirmed this. Maureen Jensen, a researcher at Harvard, and her colleagues took 98 people without back pain and did MRIs on all of them. Amazingly, she found that 36 of these subjects had significant abnormalities in their back.[23] This provided the startling information that you can have a bulging or a herniated disk in your back without pain. The converse is also true. We know very well that you can experience pain without having any detectable abnormalities in your back. You can also have pain and abnormalities in your back without the pain being due to the abnormalities.

Recently, Aaron Filler and his associates, working with 239 patients with sciatica but without any detectable ailment in the back itself, found that they could visualize piriformis syndrome with images, going down through the buttock and identifying the places where the sciatic nerve became swollen, or pressure against it increased. This process uses an MRI technique known as neuroimaging, in which standard MRI pictures are enhanced with computer software. This technique not only verifies that piriformis syndrome is present, it localizes the exact point along the course of the sciatic nerve where the compression is occurring. These special MRIs were often repeated fifteen to thirty times in each patient while administering injections and treating the patients in other ways, including surgery. The results of the research using these special MRIs are clear.

Dr. Filler and his associates provide evidence suggesting that piriformis syndrome accounts for two-thirds of the cases of sciatica that are not related to damage in the spine. In addition, the team that did this study found that more than a million cases of sciatica were not associated with a herniated disk. According to this research, nonspinal sciatica is actually more common than sciatica that is linked to a herniated disk.

CT SCAN: WHAT IT IS

The CT scan, developed in 1972, was the first computerized diagnostic imaging technique to show the inside of the body in minute cross sections, or tomographs. This scan, which utilizes X-rays, "slices" the body like a salami every millimeter or two in order to show exactly what's going on at each level.

Because the scan shows only bone and major blood vessels (without injected dye), it cannot reveal the presence, size, spatial location, and extent of tumors, blood clots, blood vessel defects, and problems in the nerves and muscles. However, the three-dimensional images can show problems in bony structures, including vertebral disks and complex joints. When it comes to the lower back, the CT allows easy access to the spinal canal, showing how wide or narrow it is, how close together the different parts of each vertebra are, and any changes in bone size, shape, or position.

Because the CT scan doesn't outline softer structures such as nerves, it doesn't reveal whether a nerve is being compressed, though a physician can come to probable conclusions from studying the formation and juxtaposition of the bones between which the nerves pass. I find that whereas the CT scan gives information that suggests a herniated disk, an MRI actually shows it, because an MRI visualizes nerve roots, disks, and other structures in good detail. The CT scan is also good for finding spinal stenosis—where it is an actual narrowing of the spinal canal— because it can measure the actual width of the canal. A CT scan is also quite useful for locating a fracture and for identifying osteoarthritis and its details, and for diagnosing spondylolisthesis. For piriformis syndrome, sacroiliac joint derangement, or musculoskeletal problems, the only advantage of a CT scan is it can reveal that none of the other maladies that might produce the same symptoms are present. It can't provide a visual image of those conditions at all.

X-RAY

X-rays have the ability to pass through matter, but how easily they do this varies with different substances. Wood and flesh are easily penetrated; denser substances such as lead and bone are more opaque. The penetrating power of X-rays also depends on their energy. The more penetrating X-rays, known as hard X-rays, are of higher frequency and are more energetic; the less penetrating X-rays, called soft X-rays, have lower energy. X-rays that have passed through a body provide a visual image of its interior structure when they strike a photographic plate or a fluorescent screen; the darkness of the shadows produced on the plate or screen depends on the relative opacity of the different parts of the body.

BONE SCAN

A bone scan shows the repair of a fracture or tumor, and arthritis and other problems. A non-toxic dose of radioactive material is injected into the bloodstream before the scan is done. As the blood circulates, particles of this material attach to cells that make up the bone. The scan is done more than once, because the radioactive material attaches to some sites quickly, and to others after an hour or two. A bone scan is different from a bone density scan, which tests only for osteoporosis.

Chapter V

CONDITIONS THAT CAUSE SCIATICA

HERNIATED DISK (HERNIATED NUCLEUS PULPOSIS)

A herniated disk (your doctor or friends might call it a "pinched nerve," "slipped disk," "ruptured disk," "bulging disk," even "sciatica") is probably the first thing people think of in connection with back pain and sciatica. (See illustration on page 56.) The very words "slipped" or "ruptured disk" conjure up images of a person lying on the floor, in pain and unable to move, waiting for an ambulance to take him or her to the operating room.

There's no question that a herniated disk may be painful, and it may injure a nerve root to the point of paralysis. People do have surgery for this problem. Until now, a herniated disk has been thought to be the most common cause of sciatica, but new data suggest that this may not be correct. The study done by Aaron Filler, et al., in 2005[24] quoted earlier studies of the MRIs of 1.2 million back pain patients nationwide and found that only 200,000 of these patients—less than 20 percent—had a herniated disk.

Still, herniated disk is a frequent occurrence, and many thousands of surgeries to correct this problem are done each year.

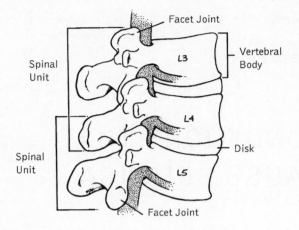

The spine's twenty-six moving parts provide a great deal of mobility. Nevertheless, there are narrow clearances for the nerves that exit at every one of them. Arthritis, swollen ligaments, herniated disks and bony narrowing can compress the nerves and cause pain. Reducing the range of motion at any joint puts additional strain on those above and below it. Increasing the range gives a margin of safety and ease.

UNDERSTANDING THE BASIC ANATOMY OF THE SPINE

All creatures with bones have a spine, and all spines are flexible. That is their virtue and why we have them. The rigidity that bones give the body, although useful, can also be a tremendous handicap when we are called upon to be flexible. The upright human being is a particularly vivid example of something called a tensegrity structure. Take a ride in the country and look at a rural radio station antenna standing alone except for the help of guy wires, which are actually pulling downward. How paradoxical that wires pulling downward should hold up the radio antenna. But that's exactly the way our muscles hold up our spine. Of course the antenna is not as jointed as our spine, and therefore our muscles are doing a far more complex job, but the analogy goes a little further. Suppose a strong wind comes along. Is the antenna likely to be stronger with tiny threads holding it steady or with a number of good solid cables? The same thing is true of our bodies. The stronger the muscles, the better our ability to remain erect.

The rigidity of bones, although amazingly effective for generating strength, leverage, and speed, are not as well suited to the versatility and flexibility demanded for survival in a three-dimensional world. The many-jointed spine must give, pitch, and twist in all three planes. At the same time it must serve as a protective conduit for transmission of information and as shock absorber of many bumps and jolts for the joints. Spinal bending can be done in the front-back plane, as in a horse galloping or humans in the process of mating. Some spines bend chiefly from side to side, including those of snakes and fish. For mankind, movement takes place in all three planes, with rotation (the most stressful and potentially injurious), especially in sports involving a ball.

The contour of the spine gives it resilience and willowy strength. The "moving parts" of the spinal column are S shaped and consist of three regions, from top to bottom: the cervical, the thoracic, and the lumbar. Along the spine are twenty-four vertebrae—doughnut-shaped bones with a tough, flexible disk between each. (See illustration on page 56.) The vertebrae are attached to one another by ligaments, tendons, and muscles. Nerves run through the spinal column, transmitting messages up to the brain and down to the arms and legs. And, more important for this discussion, nerve rootlets and nerves exit the spine on both sides through tiny openings, called neuroforamina, between each pair of vertebrae. It doesn't take much to interfere with these tiny nerve filaments, some of which descend the entire length of the spine—about 18 inches in an average adult.

The cervical spine (C1-C7), from the base of the skull to the top of the rib cage, carries the weight of the head and is extremely flexible, allowing the head to rotate, to bend to either side, and to have considerable range of movement up and down. This part of the spine is well suited to afford maximum versatility and opportunity to direct our organs of sense.

The thoracic vertebrae (T1–T12) have a much more limited range of motion, because their attachment to the ribs and sternum tethers them to one another. Whereas the curve of the cervical spine is a backward C shape, called a lordotic curve, the thoracic spine curves the other way, slightly concave, a forward curve that is referred to as kyphotic or gibbous, because of its anatomical similarity to a hump. The lumbar spine (including vertebrae numbered L1–L5) extends from the lowest part of the chest, at the level of the last rib, down to the sacrum. The lumbar spine arches backward again, like the cervical spine, in a lordotic curve. Below the lumbar spine is the sacrum, on which the lumbar spine rests. The sacrum is a single large bone consisting of five vertebrae (S1–S5) that are fused together at birth. The sacroiliac joints (another common location for back problems) connect the sacrum and pelvis on both sides. Below the sacrum is the last structure of the spine, the coccyx. It is another amalgamated bone, like the sacrum, in which four vertebrae have fused. The coccyx, often thought of as a rudimentary tail, can be injured by blunt trauma such as a fall backward.

DISKS

The disks between each pair of vertebrae are rubbery white objects that flexibly separate the vertebrae sufficiently for nerve roots to exit the inside of the vertebral column between them. In the sacrum and coccyx, there are paired openings in the solid bone through which nerve roots emerge, but past the embryonic stage there is no overt sign of disks having been there, and there is no intervertebral mobility. There is also no disk between the first vertebra and the base of the skull.

When you lift heavy groceries, jog for exercise, or twist as you hit a tennis ball, your spine is buffeted by immense outside forces. One critical function of the disks between your vertebrae is to keep the vertebrae apart, to permit the nerve roots to exit and to help hold the spine together with their strong connective tissue. The disks also act as cushions and shock absorbers, protecting the vertebrae from damage and helping the spine withstand the pressures, stresses, and strains you generate.

The disk itself is made of a tough outer layer called the annulus fibrosus. Inside, a gelatin-like substance composed partially of collagen makes up the nucleus pulposis, or center. The nucleus pulposis is viscid and pillowy; the younger you are, the plumper it is. One reason the disk may be more vulnerable as a person ages is that, as the years go by, the water content of the nucleus pulposis decreases, flattening it and reducing its ability to act as a cushion. Without the abundant fluid inside, the disk is less supple and flexible. It is more likely that the outer layer will bulge permanently or even crack (herniation), allowing some of what is inside to escape.

When herniation occurs, some portion of the disk itself moves into the canal where the nerves pass and becomes lodged in places it wasn't meant to occupy. Whether it is the hard surface of the disk or the gelatinous material inside, once it is in the tightly limited and unchangeable space of the vertebral canal, or impinging on the bony openings through which nerve roots exit the canal, it may press against and squeeze other structures (often nerves), causing inflammation, swelling, and pain. The pain may come just from the mechanical pressure of the disk part against the nerve root, or from the inflammation and swelling that irritate and further crowd an already tight space, raising pressure still further in the fixed confines of the spinal canal.

Most disk herniations occur in the bottom two disks in the lumbar spine, between L4 and L5, or between L5 and S1, though herniation may occur at any level. Herniated disks can cause either of two conditions associated with sciatica, depending on where the disk material goes after the herniation. One condition is radiculopathy, in which the neuroforamina—the small openings through which nerve roots exit the spinal canal—are narrowed. Radiculopathy is a common medical term that your doctor is likely to use if you have a herniated disk. The second condition is called spinal stenosis, a reduction of the space inside the canal itself, which may affect multiple nerve roots that pass by that level. It is possible to have a radiculopathy *and* spinal stenosis.

The most common cause of a herniated disk is lifting something too heavy. Overuse, or lifting something that isn't too heavy but lifting it over and over again, is the second most common situation that I see in connection with a herniated disk. Just the way a metal coat hanger fatigues and finally breaks apart if bent in the same place too many times, a disk that is regularly displaced from its natural position will also tend to crack its annulus fibrosus and allow nucleus pulposis material to push out and into the space behind it, where the nerve roots conduct messages from the brain to the body and back again.

Twisting movements, especially while carrying something heavy—for example, moving an old, heavy computer monitor from one desk to another—can cause a herniated disk. Injury can occur from staying too long in an uncomfortable position—for example, sitting in a tiny car for hours. A trauma—including a fall, a blow on the head, an automobile accident, or anything else that applies sudden and focal force—can injure a disk. Sometimes, without any apparent reason, a disk just herniates. People sometimes go to bed at night feeling fine and wake up in the morning with a herniated disk. Frequently no specific cause can be identified.

SYMPTOMS, SIGNS, AND DIAGNOSIS OF HERNIATED DISK

A herniated disk, like sciatica, is usually accompanied by some degree of back pain and stiffness. There is usually muscle spasm. Often the person feels weakness, numbness, or tingling as well. A herniated disk may be more painful on one side than the other. The pain may be sharp. Whereas the classic signs of sciatica are the feeling of electric shocks along the course of the nerve: in the buttock, the back of the thigh, the back and outside of the calf, the heel, the space between the first and second toes, the outside of the top of the foot, and/or the sole of the foot, if you have a herniated disk you may also feel unpleasant symptoms on the surface of the skin, including pins and needles, hot and cold, and "ants crawling."

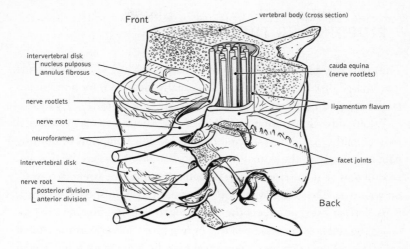

The spine is a busy place, combining strength to support the body and protect the nerves, and flexibility to enable the body to bend for action and bounce back from trauma.

MYTHS ABOUT HERNIATED DISK

Does a herniated disk always mean pain and sciatica? Definitely not. We have already quoted Maureen Jensen's classic study, which suggested that more than 30 percent of people who don't have any backache whatsoever do have abnormalities in their vertebral disks.[25] And we have also mentioned the 1.2 million MRIs that found only 200,000 of these patients, less than 20 percent, had herniated disks. Therefore, if you do have sciatic-type pain, it is possible that the pain is not coming from a herniated disk, even if you *do* have one! Nor does a herniated disk absolutely lead to early surgery. We have found that 80 to 90 percent of these "slipped disks" may be handled outside a hospital, with conservative treatments. If pain continues unabated for more than three to six weeks, or worsens significantly, surgery may be indicated.

PINPOINTING THE PROBLEM

The connection between the nature of the symptoms and the location of a herniated disk at the spinal level is usually clear and, for a physician familiar with the patient's anatomy, relatively easy to read.

When a disk herniation occurs at L5-S1, the injury may produce a radiculopathy. Tingling, pins and needles, and/or numbness or burning pain may occur on the skin of the outer calf and/or between the first and second toes or at the heel. It may be difficult to find the strength to walk on your toes. The Achilles tendon reflex may be diminished or absent.

A herniation that affects the nerve root(s) at L4-L5 generally produces the tingling, pins and needles, or numbness and/or burning pain at the inner calf or along the instep. Weakness shows up in walking on your heels or "footdrop." A reflex that is often difficult to elicit even in the normal leg—striking the anterior tibial tendon (the big tendon in front of your ankle bone) to cause the foot to rise toward the shin—may be affected by this. But inability to elicit this reflex is nothing to worry about. A lot of physicians can't do it either.

When the problem is at L3-L4, the numbness or other sensory complaints are centered around the knee and the front of the thigh. Weakness of the quadriceps may impede walking up or down stairs, or cause the knees to buckle. The patellar tendon reflex (the "knee jerk" reflex) may be feeble or absent.

At L2-L3, the weakness may be the same, involving difficulty with straightening the knee, or it may appear as weakened adduction—difficulty in bringing and holding the legs together, especially while they're bearing the body's weight. The symptoms—the tingling, pins and needles, burning, and pain—are often located farther up the thigh. There is no reflex that doctors usually check here, but one of the adductor muscles (which bring the thighs together) would be appropriate.

At L1-L2, the sensations of pain, numbness, tingling, and the rest are not in the front of the thigh but much more often at the inner or outer thigh. Weakness is in flexing the thigh—bringing it up in front of you

NERVE ROOT SYMPTOMS CHART

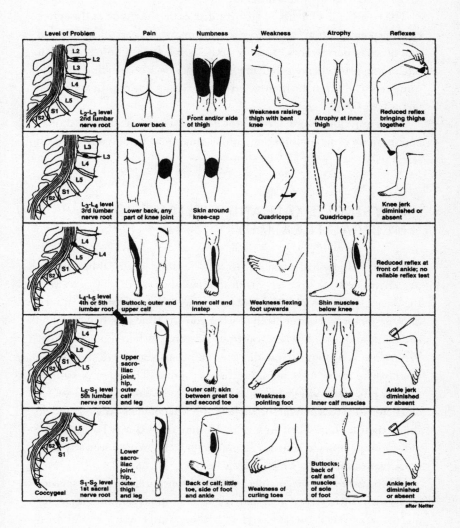

Level of Problem	Pain	Numbness	Weakness	Atrophy	Reflexes
L2-L3 level 2nd lumbar nerve root	Lower back	Front and/or side of thigh	Weakness raising thigh with bent knee	Atrophy at inner thigh	Reduced reflex bringing thighs together
L3-L4 level 3rd lumbar nerve root	Lower back, any part of knee joint	Skin around knee-cap	Quadriceps	Quadriceps	Knee jerk diminished or absent
L4-L5 level 4th or 5th lumbar root	Buttock; outer and upper calf	Inner calf and instep	Weakness flexing foot upwards	Shin muscles below knee	Reduced reflex at front of ankle; no reliable reflex test
L5-S1 level 5th lumbar nerve root	Upper sacro-iliac joint, hip, outer calf and leg	Outer calf; skin between great toe and second toe	Weakness pointing foot	inner calf muscles	Ankle jerk diminished or absent
S1-S2 level 1st sacral nerve root Coccygeal	Lower sacro-iliac joint, hip, outer thigh and leg	Back of calf; little toe, side of foot and ankle	Weakness of curling toes	Buttocks; back of calf and muscles of sole of foot	Ankle jerk diminished or absent

after Netter

Here is a way to home-diagnose the level of your herniated disk.

like a drum major. Striking the iliopsoas muscle in the lateral groin (near the middle of your front pants pocket) might show asymmetrically less response on the side that is affected.

The herniation of a disk so that it intrudes on the inside of the spinal canal produces spinal stenosis, or narrowing, which can affect fibers of one or more nerve roots, possibly on both sides of the spine. There is often more pain when you're lying flat on your back or standing with the spine relatively straight than when you're sitting down, or lying curled up on your side.

The symptoms I've described for each level of herniated disk may appear alone or in combination, and at times may be different on each side.

PHYSICAL EXAM AND INITIAL MEDICAL TREATMENT

A history and physical exam in the doctor's office is critical in diagnosing a herniated disk. In every medical school they say that 90 percent of the diagnosis for any physical problem comes from the patient's history. So your doctor had better listen to what you say. How long have you had the pain, and does it wake you from sleeping? What about tingling? Where are you numb? How did the symptoms start? Are they worse when you're sitting or standing? Is there weakness? The questions go on.

Your physician will test muscle strength and weakness, and look for characteristic areas of numbness. He or she will compare reflexes, and do the straight leg test. Then an EMG, CT scan, or MRI may be ordered. If a disk problem is identified, you are likely to be treated initially with conservative measures, which usually help.

Noninvasive ways to manage a painful herniated disk and sciatica begin with cutting down your activity level to 40 percent of normal. Ice and heat, physical therapy, and over-the-counter nonsteroidal anti-inflammatory painkillers are recommended. But individuals who have a herniated disk are often in a great deal of pain, including the classic accompanying sciatica radiating down the leg (usually the worst part), and lower back pain. You may feel like going to bed and staying there. There are many differing opinions as to the appropriate level of activity for a person with a herniated disk. I believe in a moderate approach. For most of us, total rest is a novelty, and the results of it are therefore unknown. It certainly makes one stiff. Don't rest so much that you get weaker, but certainly don't be so active that you tire yourself out. Take it very easy for a week or so, then reassess. Short spurts of total bed rest may help, but four days of bed rest have been shown to worsen back pain and sciatica.[26]

Internists' first line of treatment of a herniated disk often begins with a nonsteroidal anti-inflammatory, possibly one of the older, more innocuous but still potent drugs such as Diclofenac (Voltaren.) A muscle relaxant such as metaxalone (Skelaxin) or carisoprodol (Soma) is also often prescribed. In my own practice I seldom use these two old muscle relaxants because of their surprisingly addictive properties. When appropriate I use a very low dose of cyclobenzaprine, which is significantly less sedating than many others but just as effective at lowering muscle tension. Why are muscle relaxants standard for severe back pain? Because they sometimes reduce the spasm, which is a large part of the discomfort.

Stronger and weaker oral medicines are also available. Tylenol with codeine and synthetic morphine in many combinations are often effective short-run ways to ferry people over the roughest stretch, which may come a few hours to a few weeks after injury. Tramadol (Ultram) and Lidocaine and fentanyl skin patches have claimed important places in reducing discomfort to tolerable levels and beyond.

In addition, physical therapy can do wonders for a person with a herniated disk. I have found that early intervention with McKenzie technique, myofascial work, manual medical techniques, and modalities such as heat, electrical stimulation, and ultrasound, and, where appropriate, craniosacral therapy and yoga, have taken more than 85 percent of my patients with a herniated disk out of the realm of surgical consideration, and over time have produced results that are at least as beneficial as those from surgery.

The "touching cure"—physical therapy—also provides emotional reassurance, something that a surgical team doesn't always give. In chronic cases, it also produces strategic anatomically based approaches to long-term pain relief. In an overwhelmingly large number of patients I have treated, I have seen that three hours a week of physical therapy at the onset of an episode of sciatica shortens the duration of the attack, lessens its severity, and reduces the likelihood of recurrence.[27]

PIRIFORMIS SYNDROME

Sciatica is always a nerve problem relating to fibers that make up the sciatic nerve. Although it may involve damage to these and other nerve fibers in the spine, that isn't always the case. An injury in the lumbosacral plexus, just below and a little on either side of the spine, where the fibers from all the major nerves in the leg—including the sciatic nerve—are redistributed, can cause sciatica in any spot along the fibers' course. Sciatica can also be caused by cancer, tuberculosis, an abscess, a gunshot wound, multiple sclerosis, fracture, meningitis—anything that affects the neurons, which transmit messages from the nerve, or that alters the central nervous system, where reports from the sciatic nerve can be misinterpreted.

A common form of sciatica comes from a condition called piriformis syndrome, when the sciatic nerve becomes entrapped and squeezed as it passes below the piriformis muscle. In the vast majority of cases, piriformis syndrome occurs when the piriformis muscle in the buttock compresses the sciatic nerve, pushing it against the sharp, tendon-like structures that lie beneath it. (See illustrations on pages 67 and 68.) I estimate that about 90 percent of the time, this syndrome begins when the piriformis muscle goes into spasm. The resulting nerve compression causes sciatica.

What does it feel like? Well, it has often been described as "a royal pain in the butt." But it can go further, including pain in the hip and up in the lumbar region and, yes, sciatica all the way down the leg. People who have piriformis syndrome may frustrate their physicians, because it can be hard to diagnose. Results of MRIs and standard EMGs look completely normal. Many of the people struck by this syndrome are healthy.

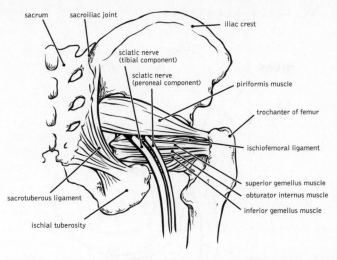

Generally the sciatic nerve passes just beneath the piriformis muscle, and above the sharp edge of the ischiofemoral ligament and the superior gemellus muscle.

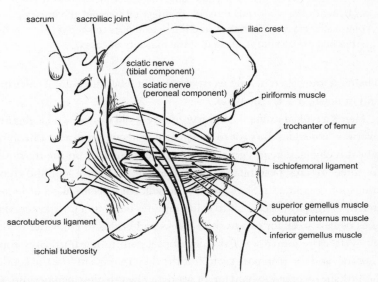

Approximately 15 percent of the time, one or both divisions of the sciatic nerve pass through the piriformis muscle. Although this is generally unrelated to piriformis syndrome, it does complicate surgery, which is essential about 0.4 percent of the time.

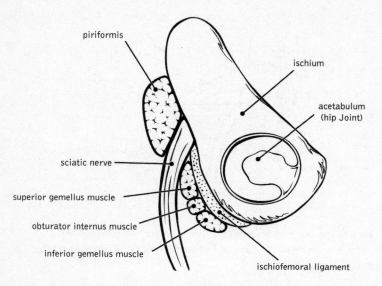

piriformis

ischium

acetabulum
(hip Joint)

sciatic nerve

superior gemellus muscle

obturator internus muscle

inferior gemellus muscle

ischiofemoral ligament

A side view shows just how vulnerable the sciatic nerve is as it passes beneath the piriformis muscle. An injection to quiet the muscle, physical therapy to stretch it, and home exercises to keep it stretched are all that is needed in the majority of cases.

The more they exercise, the worse it gets, but when they stop exercising and sit down, it gets still worse.

Here's a typical example. A thirty-five-year-old woman who is slightly overweight decides she's got to do something about her fitness. She joins a health club and begins going there regularly, running on the treadmill for three minutes, pushing to increase her stamina. Pretty soon she's running for forty minutes. She's proud of herself, but it seems like a little too much, so she pulls back a bit to thirty minutes but runs a little faster. She goes twice a week for two to three weeks and begins to enjoy her workout. After the fourth week she develops a pain in her butt. She stops running, and the pain goes away. But she doesn't want to lose the conditioning she's worked so hard for, or waste her health club membership, so she starts running again after a few days. The pain returns, this time so severely that she has to leave the treadmill and sit down. But when she sits down, the pain—instead of going away—actually becomes worse.

The scenario can also go like this. A man is playing tennis, increasing the time he puts in, getting in better and better condition. But sometimes he feels something he wouldn't even describe as pain. It's just a funny feeling at the outside of the calf, the back of the thigh, or the top of the foot. The trouble is, it gets worse, and it gets much worse when he's sitting around waiting for the next set. It feels really bad when he has to climb the stairs or go up a hill, and it's almost terrible when he does a general fitness session, with squats. Sometimes all these symptoms are accompanied by weakness, preventing him from walking on tiptoe, and causing feeble reflexes, numbness in all his toes, even impotence.

Although these cases are typical, a fall or other trauma can also cause piriformis syndrome. You can sustain a blow by falling backward on the stairs. That's one I've come across quite often. The injury can come from an automobile accident in which you were hit from behind. More unusual but possible is being overweight to the point that the fat wads up at your buttock when you sit in such a way that it actually compresses the nerve.

Sitting for long periods of time, especially in a car or on an airplane, can also cause this painful condition, which can become chronic. Any event that can put the piriformis muscle in spasm, making it clench tightly enough to affect the nerve, can cause this problem.

OVERUSE AND OTHER CAUSES OF PIRIFORMIS SYNDROME

The most common cause of piriformis syndrome is overuse. That's what happened to the woman on the treadmill and the tennis enthusiast. Other sports can also cause overuse injury, especially basketball and backpacking. One of my patients told me, "I've been walking up that hill since I was eleven years old—nearly sixty years. It can't be bad for me." Of course for this gentleman, it was overuse, because his age and other problems had led to a general weakening of all his muscles, making the piriformis muscle more vulnerable to injury. The hill did not change. What changed was his capacity to climb it.

Sitting for long periods may fall into the category of overuse. This is a common cause of piriformis syndrome that affects computer users, commuters, bus drivers, psychiatrists, bankers, secretaries, and many others, even vacationers who spend a long time in transit.

Sprain or strain can also cause piriformis syndrome. Pulling a recalcitrant weed out of the garden can do it. Almost falling but catching yourself before you fall by putting your foot in the wrong place may apply so much leverage that you overstretch the muscle. You can do it by reaching for a heavy iron pot on the back burner.

The American Running Association lists the following causes of piriformis syndrome:

* Muscle spasms
* Overtraining
* Biomechanics (including leg length differences)
* Muscle imbalances (such as the abdomen and quadriceps not being strong enough to work properly with hamstrings and lower back muscles)
* Prolonged sitting (which puts too much pressure on the piriformis muscle)
* Poor stretching (tight hip flexors can put too much pressure on the piriformis muscle, irritating the sciatic nerve)[28]

PIRIFORMIS SYNDROME DOES EXIST

Piriformis syndrome is common, and it's difficult. Over a 16-year period, I saw 6,000 patients who had piriformis syndrome in my New York office. These patients had been suffering from sciatica for an average of 6.2 years and had seen an average of 6.5 clinicians before they came to me. Among them, they had had thousands of MRIs, X-rays, and surgeries while searching for a diagnosis and cure. But at the time, few people knew what they should be looking for (nerve entrapment in the buttock), let alone how to find it.

Not only is piriformis syndrome widespread and problematic, it is

controversial. Some doctors believe that it's significant and underdiagnosed; others believe that it doesn't even exist, that it should never be
diagnosed or treated. At the turn of the century in the United States,
some physicians said that piriformis syndrome was caused by arthritis;
others thought it was irritation of the nerve by tuberculosis or bursitis.
The latter were on the right track about nerve irritation, of course, but
they didn't identify the piriformis muscle as the culprit. Some people
have since written that piriformis syndrome has vascular causes; others
have asserted that it's an anatomical anomaly in the way the nerve and
muscle relate to each other.

As recently as 2003, the National Institute of Neurological Disorders
and Stroke described piriformis syndrome as "a rare neuromuscular disorder." And the National Institutes of Health has defined it away by
declaring that sciatica is an "injury to the sciatic nerve fibers in the lumbar spine."[29] *Stedman's Medical Dictionary* (25th edition; Baltimore,
Maryland: Williams & Wilkins, 1982) defines sciatica as " . . . pain in
the lower back and hip radiating down the back of the thigh into the
leg, usually due to lumbar disk." This, at least, leaves some room for piriformis syndrome. Linking this problem with low back pain, researchers
at Weill Medical College of Cornell University found that piriformis
syndrome could constitute up to 5 percent of cases of low back, buttock,
and leg pain.[30] Even this would mean that as many as 4 million people
are afflicted with piriformis syndrome each year.

Knowing how common piriformis syndrome is and acknowledging
that it really does exist and is a significant health problem is a continuing dilemma. "True incidence of piriformis is not clear at this time,"
Aaron Filler and his colleagues wrote in a superb paper published in
2005. "Lacking agreement even on the existence of the diagnosis and
how to establish if it does exist, epidemiological work has been scarce."
Filler, et al., cite a study that we have already mentioned of 1.2 million
MRIs done on people with sciatica that found only 200,000 of them
with "treatable herniated disk." Filler's conclusion is a stunning one for
those who might have been in doubt about piriformis syndrome: "One
interpretation of the results obtained in our study population is that piriformis syndrome may be as common as herniated disks in the cause of

sciatica."[31] Still, I believe that many physicians, physicians' assistants, and other health professionals are unaware or only vaguely aware of it.

My colleagues and I began modern methods of diagnosis of piriformis syndrome using the H-reflex and EMG in 1987.[32] We timed the H-reflex of normal subjects in the position of flexion, adduction, and internal rotation (the FAIR-test). In that position the piriformis muscle tightly presses the sciatic nerve against the underlying structures. After that a comparison was made; we compared the timing with the H-reflex in the normal position with the timing in the FAIR position. There was essentially no change.

However, things were different in sciatica patients without clinical evidence of a herniated disk or any other spinal abnormality, pain with pressure on or in the buttock where the sciatic nerve goes under the piriformis muscle, and pain and/or weakness with the patient resisting abduction of the flexed thigh.

In a great majority of these patients, the H-reflex was slowed by more than three standard deviations—something that would statistically occur by chance less than once in a hundred trials in people with no back pain. And it was delayed when the test was repeated multiple times. (See graph on page 73.)

Patients who met the clinical criteria for piriformis syndrome exhibited this delay. Almost twenty years ago, I published an abstract of a clinical trial in which we identified patients meeting the clinical criteria for piriformis syndrome by using this method.[33] Fortunately for those who have piriformis syndrome, more people believe in it now than did then.

My first piriformis syndrome patient was an operating room nurse at a hospital in the Bronx. Her imaging tests showed no problems, yet sciatica on both sides troubled her. Her orthopedic surgeon told me he thought she had some difficulty with her sciatic nerve. At the time I knew how to identify a herniated disk, but the surgeon reiterated that it hurt only when the patient was sitting down. Sometimes her pain also flared up when she had been standing too long. I wanted to help with a diagnosis, but I didn't know of a test for something like that. The surgeon said, "Do something functional." Then he looked at his watch, told me he was late for his next appointment, and left.

H-Reflexes

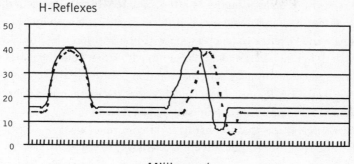

Milliseconds

The time it takes to complete the H-reflex in the anatomical position is compared to the H-reflex time in flexion, adduction, and internal rotation of the leg (FAIR-test), which will compress the sciatic nerve if the patient has piriformis syndrome. If the FAIR-test delays the H-reflex more than three standard deviations beyond the mean, we have a diagnosis.

Utility of the FAIR-Test

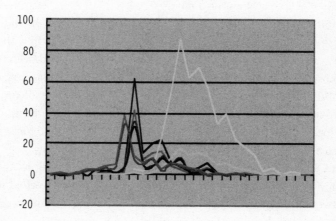

People with symptoms of piriformis syndrome are easily distinguished from normal individuals using the FAIR-test.

I thought of comparing the H-reflex on one side with the other, but this patient had a problem on both sides. Then it came to me. I could compare the H-reflex in one position with the position that brought on pain. It didn't take long and didn't hurt much. When I put the patient in the flexion, adduction, and internal rotation position—what came to be known as the FAIR-test—I saw evidence that the surgeon was right: the patient's sciatic nerve was significantly compressed.

The surgeon was glad to hear it, for it confirmed what he suspected. When he took her to her surgery a few days later, I went with them, snapping photos during the operation to show residents who had never seen anything like this before. It was all too clear. During the surgery, we saw that just below the gluteus maximus, the outermost muscle in the buttock, was the piriformis muscle, glistening and sharp. Beneath that was the sciatic nerve, where the little blood vessels that generally serve the nerve itself had been obliterated near the area where the muscle crossed it. The damage was not subtle.

It was an "aha" moment for the surgeon. He thinned the muscle down by perhaps 20 percent, instilled steroid to reduce any inflammatory reaction, then sewed the patient back up. She was in some pain for a few days, but it was clear that we had gotten to the cause, and the surgeon had been able to accomplish a repair.

That was when I decided to see if the FAIR-test brought the same results with "normals" too. When I saw that it didn't, I knew that we were on to something. Until then, piriformis syndrome had been only a diagnosis of exclusion—that is, a diagnosis made only after every other possibility was ruled out. Later, as my skills and those of my staff improved and we understood more about this painful condition, we developed a physical therapy protocol that did so much good for so many patients that surgery for this problem is rather unusual today.

In Olmsted County, Minnesota, home of the Mayo Clinic, the frequency of diagnosis of piriformis syndrome has gone up fivefold in the last twenty-five years. The Walter Reed Hospital in Washington, D.C., confirmed slightly higher levels in 2001.

As I see it, the vast majority of physicians are uninformed, misinformed, or underinformed about piriformis syndrome. Most of the practitioners who do concern themselves with the workings and interactions between muscles and nerves—the orthopedic surgeons, physical therapists, chiropractors, osteopaths, and doctors of physical medicine and rehabilitation—are aware of the condition and the treatment for it.

HOME DIAGNOSIS OF PIRIFORMIS SYNDROME

If you're wondering whether you have piriformis syndrome, you can do a lot to diagnose yourself at home. First, is the pain worse when you're sitting down? Do you have pain, numbness, and/or weakness in the buttock, down the back of the leg, or both? Without such discomfort, you can rule out piriformis syndrome. Next, if you press on the muscle in each buttock, just a little above the middle of the cheek, and you have pain on one side or both sides, that is another indication that you have piriformis syndrome. Sometimes you can feel the muscle in spasm there. If you don't feel any pain, tenderness, or discomfort with this pressure, chances are you don't have the problem, though I've seen a few exceptions to this rule. Third, the straight leg raise test, discussed on page 40, should cause more pain on the side that is affected by piriformis syndrome when the leg is held at a lower angle than on the other side.

Here are some specifics for performing the FAIR-test at home. This simpler version of the test, developed by a Norwegian surgeon named Solheim, is done without an EMG machine. Although the test is not definitive, it might help you figure out what's wrong. The Solheim test and the Pace's test (below) are easier with a friend.

Lie on your side on the floor, with the painful side up. Bring the knee of the leg on that side down to the floor, without turning over and without facing downward. A friend can do that part and the next. Now press your knee downward and move the ankle upward, more or less using the leg as a crank to turn the hip joint counterclockwise (on the left) and clockwise (on the right). If you feel pain, you may well have piriformis syndrome.

There is also Pace's test, which takes a partner to complete. Assume the

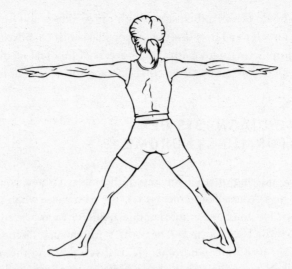

The Twisted Triangle pose helps treat piriformis syndrome. Face the wall and twist away from it.

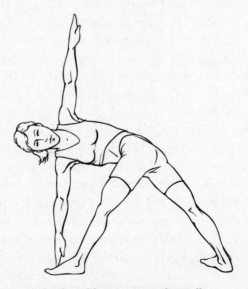

After twisting, rest your back and hips against the wall.

MY SAMPLE PRESCRIPTION FOR
PIRIFORMIS SYNDROME*

1. Place patient in contralateral decubitus and flexed, adducted, internally rotated (FAIR) position.**

2. Ultrasound applied to piriformis muscle while leg is placed in flexion, adduction, and internal rotation (FAIR) position: 2.25 to 2.5 watts/cm^2 for 10 to 14 minutes. Beware of patients with any hypoesthesia or anesthesia due to neurological or surgical causes in the dorsal lumbosacral region. Physical therapists, beware of cavitation in post-laminectomy patients.***

3. Wipe off ultrasound gel.

4. Apply hot packs or cold spray at the same location for 10 minutes.

5. Stretch the piriformis muscle for 10 to 14 minutes by applying manual pressure to the muscle's inferior border, being careful not to press downward; instead, direct the pressure tangentially, toward the ipsilateral shoulder.****

6. Myofascial release at the lumbosacral paraspinal muscles.

7. McKenzie exercises.

8. Use a lumbosacral corset when the patient is in the FAIR position.*****

Duration: 2 to 3 times weekly for 1 to 2 months.

* Patients usually require 2 to 3 months of biweekly therapy for 50 to 70 percent improvement.
** Because the FAIR-position may be painful, patients often subtly shift to prone. This must be avoided, because it places the affected leg in abduction, not adduction, greatly reducing the stretch placed on the piriformis muscle.
*** Cavitation is unreported in more than 20,000 treatments.
**** Unless explicitly stated, therapists should not knead or massage the muscle, which is useless or worse. The muscle must be stretched perpendicular to its fibers, in a plane that would be tangent to the buttock at the point of intersection of the piriformis muscle and the sciatic nerve, but approximately 3/4 inch deep into the buttock (that is, just below the gluteus maximus).
***** This is useful in patients who have had a laminectomy, or in others to prevent lumbar hypermobility.

same position (see illustration on page 37). Raise your bent leg. Your friend should try earnestly but not too vigorously to keep it down. Once your leg is up in the air, hold it there. If you're weaker on one side than the other, that's another indication that you may be suffering from piriformis syndrome. Get the full FAIR-test if there are any abnormalities.

A conventional X-ray will not show piriformis syndrome, nor will any standard MRI or EMG. However, the spasm of the piriformis muscle can affect the sciatic nerve and can damage or even sever some of its fibers, and an EMG *can* pick up that damage.

The various types of exertion that could have caused the piriformis syndrome in the first place can also make it worse, or make it begin again if it has eased up. Running on a treadmill is an example of this, as is walking up steep stairs or a hill, or heavy lifting for a long period of time.

Most of the time, people who have piriformis syndrome have it on one side only, but I have seen individuals who have it on one side, then get it on the other side as well. The pressure of the abnormally large or stiff piriformis muscle pulls the sciatic nerve quite taut. Women are built so that the nerve fibers that make up the sciatic nerve travel close to the side wall of the vagina, and the male organ pressing against that wall may produce pain in women who have piriformis syndrome. In fact, if the sexual act causes a woman to have sciatica, it is almost certainly caused by piriformis syndrome.

Treatment for piriformis syndrome has been refined, along with its growing recognition. Our piriformis syndrome treatment protocol for physical therapists is as follows. While lying comfortably in the FAIR position, the patient receives 2 to 2.5 watts per square centimeter of ultrasound for 10 to 14 minutes. This is applied in broad strokes longitudinally along the piriformis muscle. After the ultrasound gel is wiped off, hot packs or cold spray are placed at the same location for 10 minutes. The physical therapist uses manual pressure to help stretch the piriformis muscle (without kneading or massaging it). The pressure should be directed sideways—that is, not downward, but perpendicular to the muscle fibers in a plane that is horizontal to the buttock at the intersection of the piriformis muscle and the sciatic nerve, about 3/4 inch into the buttock, or just below the gluteus maximus muscle. Myofascial release at the lumbosacral paraspinal muscles is recommended, along with McKenzie exercises. Patients who have had laminectomy, fusion, or spondylolisthesis should wear a lumbosacral corset when being treated in the FAIR position.

We recommend physical therapy two or three times a week for one to three months. We have also recommended ten specific yoga poses in our book *Cure Back Pain with Yoga*. Two poses are pictured on page 76.

SPINAL STENOSIS: WHAT IT IS

Stenosis means narrowing. To understand spinal stenosis, it's necessary to make the distinction between two types of openings: one in the neuroforamina and the other in the spinal canal itself. The neuroforamina are the little openings between the vertebrae at which the nerve rootlets consolidate into roots and through which they exit the spine like the branches of a Christmas tree leaving the trunk—symmetrically on both sides. The fibers in those nerve roots are destined to descend to the lumbosacral plexus, where they combine, divide, and recombine to form the peripheral nerves, including the sciatic nerve. When these little neuroforaminal openings are narrowed because of swelling, irritation, or some other problem, the result is a radiculopathy: pain and possibly sciatica, but not spinal stenosis. For example, if the nerve roots that come out of the neuroforamina at L4-L5 are compressed because they don't have enough space, you will feel it on the skin inside your calf, and the ability to lift your foot at your ankle will be compromised as a specific consequence of injury to a specific nerve root.

Spinal stenosis is narrowing within the spinal canal itself. If that happens and you have compression at the same level that I described above, it could affect the same nerves with the same feelings, the same weaknesses. After all, the same nerve fibers are involved; it's just that they're injured at a slightly different place. But there's a distinction. If the problem is in the neuroforamen, it's just one nerve that is injured. But if it's the central canal, it could easily affect nerves on both sides below it, at L5-S1 and any and all nerves below that. That's a big difference. The symptoms may be different. When you have a single level at which an injury occurs, you have a neat package of symptoms that many physicians can recognize at once, and identify. Recognizing spinal stenosis may be a challenge.

SYMPTOMS, DIAGNOSIS, AND CAUSES

Stenosis often begins with a vague kind of discomfort over broad areas of skin, even in places that are not related to the sciatic nerve. You may feel numbness or tingling, mild or severe burning sensations at the outside of your thighs or in your calves or feet. Unlike problems with the neuroforamina, symptoms of stenosis are often bilateral—more or less symmetrical, though that doesn't mean they're always or necessarily exactly equal on both sides. Some cases of stenosis are evident on one side only. Stenosis can have a number of different manifestations. You may feel it on the inside of the arches of your feet, or inside the thighs, or just below the buttocks or knees, or a combination of these.

The reason the symptoms may be hard to pin down is that swelling inside the spine is usually (but not always) progressive, and the narrowing is often a chronic and incremental process. The progression isn't smooth or linear. Today you may experience mild pain, another day it feels as though you're wearing sweat pants even though you may be wearing nothing. When stenosis is sudden, it can come from a disk that has begun to bulge or has cracked and become swollen in the middle of the spine, instead of nearer the outer edge, where it is at the neuroforamen. Nevertheless, the swelling that results may mildly compress one clump of rootlets today and another clump a week from now.

A significant feature of stenosis is that the symptoms are often worse when the spine is straight. That means you will be more uncomfortable when you're lying flat and are horizontal, or standing up and entirely vertical. Sitting with the spine somewhat curved provides some relief, as does lying in the fetal position. A simple explanation for this is that nerves are stretched more and are therefore thinner when the spine is curved. When your spine is straight, the nerves are as thick as they can get in a space that doesn't enlarge, and therefore they are more subject to compression.

If there is sciatica, but the symptoms don't fit into a neat package of a single level of spinal injury, that's another suggestion that you might have stenosis. There are ways to distinguish this problem from piriformis syndrome. First, piriformis syndrome is almost always worse when you're sitting down. Second, in spinal stenosis, pressing the buttock is painless. If there are symptoms or signs in the front of the thigh, or the inner part of the calves, it's due to an injury of fibers that are not part of the sciatic nerve. These never come close to the piriformis muscle, so piriformis syndrome is not the problem in this case.

Stenosis often distinguishes itself from most radiculopathies because pain doesn't occur at a specific place or have an abrupt beginning, and there is pain on both sides. Unlike a disk problem at the neuroforamen, this condition can interfere with all the nerve rootlets of the cauda equina below it. The nerves that control the sphincters of the bowel and bladder can be affected. If you feel ascending numbness or weakness, or if you have issues with bowel and bladder control, that is a medical emergency and requires immediate attention. Very unusual, sudden, and severe lumbar spinal stenosis can cause cauda equina syndrome, and limit voluntary control of all muscles and sphincters below it.

To be absolutely certain that your problem is stenosis, you will need an MRI. This diagnostic test can determine the size of the space inside the spinal canal and can outline the soft tissue inside it, such as the ligamentum flavum and the nerves. The EMG is the gold standard of measuring how much damage there is, and at what levels it has occurred. A myelogram or the injection of X-ray contrast fluid by a radiologist is also useful in showing the exact location and nature of any compression. It is done in conjunction with an X-ray or CT scan, often before surgery is performed.

Spinal stenosis most often results from a gradual, degenerative aging process, but not always. Three elements precipitate this condition. A cross section of the spinal column at any level from the top to the bottom always contains the same elements: the bony sides of the canal; the disks, which separate the vertebral bodies at the front of the canal; and the ligamentum flavum (the yellow ligament), which lines the back of the canal continuously from the neck down. Stenosis comes about when one or more of these elements bulges or herniates into the canal, narrowing it enough to put pressure on the nerve fibers within it.

This reduced diameter occurs most often and predictably when osteoarthritis and similar processes thicken the bones. When you're young, your bones get longer; with age, they get thicker, and the spaces within the bone become narrower. (See illustration on page 61.)

If the ligamentum flavum thickens, the space available for the nervous tissue is decreased by the same amount. Although age and chronic, gradual processes such as osteoarthritis are generally responsible for bony thickening, it is an abrupt event or a short-term situation such as sleeping in an unnatural position on a cramped couch for a couple of hours that can cause the ligamentum flavum to swell and constrict the available space.

Disks bulge and herniate for all kinds of reasons—from lifting firewood and reaching for the turkey platter while serving a large gathering, to falls, overuse, and awkward movements in restless sleep. Whereas the bony changes and ligamentum flavum thickening can occur throughout a large sector of the spine, disk-related narrowing is usually located at one particular level.

The illustration on page 61 makes it clear that a significant enlargement in any of these three elements is no more serious than mild or moderate enlargement in two or three of them. Yet the remedies for the three are quite different. We'll get to that later. For now, we've characterized spinal stenosis, and gotten familiar with its causes.

When spinal stenosis produces pain, it's rarely explained by a single acute event. Various elements limit the space inside the spinal canal, and something happens to disturb the normal equilibrium of two of the following three elements:

* the ligamentum flavum, which stretches continuously from the neck to the sacral spine
* the disk that abuts on the cylinder at each level
* the actual diameter of the cylinder that the nerves pass through

Treatments for these situations are different. If the ligamentum flavum has become swollen, usually steroids introduced into the epidural space will reduce that swelling—until you sleep on that short couch again or do whatever you did to bring about the pain. Steroids may cure your condition forever. If it's a disk problem, steroids can be helpful here, too, in reducing the size of the disk itself and damping down the chemical reactions that often ensue from its inflammation. And that will also provide more room for the nerves. If the cause of the stenosis is due to changes in the bones, surgery is the only reliable cure. There is an exception to this, however. If you're in an acute situation, epidurals may work by narrowing other elements and reducing inflammation that the narrowing of bone has produced, at least for a few weeks. You can often buy a little time with epidural steroids.

How do you determine the cause of any particular case of stenosis? An MRI is invaluable. Neuroimaging may prove to be valuable, and in the future such techniques may be able to reveal the exact nature of an injury. Your medical history and a complete physical will also be helpful. If the condition has an abrupt onset, chances are it's not just osteoarthritis and the slow and inevitable encroachment of thickening bone into the spinal canal, but specific events that have produced bulging or herniation of a disk or swelling of the ligamentum flavum. Steroids are more likely to work in an acute event than with chronic, creeping, encroaching bone. If the symptoms are gradually increasing, if they involve the outside of your thighs, going down toward your knees and lower part of the legs, you have a chronic, progressive problem. Rather than drift into the position of an old person whose cardiovascular system will no longer tolerate an operation, without which life is either unbearable or dominated by having to take many medications, surgery is the most sensible alternative.

SPONDYLOLISTHESIS

This is another condition that affects what's going on inside the spinal column. Although it is estimated to occur in 4 to 6 percent of the general population,[34] like other back problems that show up on diagnostic tests, it is sometimes asymptomatic. At other times it causes pain, and we would estimate that in 10 percent of the cases we've seen, it results in sciatica.

In Greek, "spondy" means spine and "listhesis" means slip. When the isthmus of bone that connects the vertebral body to its four joints—two above and two below (pars interarticularis)—is damaged, the vertebral body may slide forward. This usually happens low down in the spine, at L3, L4, or L5. It can begin in childhood, and in most cases no treatment is needed. However, this condition can cause nerve compression by narrowing the neuroforamina at a single level, or by narrowing the inside of the spinal canal, which could affect all of the nerves that traverse that level and go below it. In other words, it can cause sciatica in the same ways that a herniated disk or spinal stenosis does.

Symptoms are often similar to those of herniated disk and/or spinal stenosis. There may be pain in the back, and weakness, numbness, and heaviness in the legs. Also, there is often classic nerve pain: tingling and burning and electric shocks. We frequently find that patients with tingling at the outside of the thigh, especially when arching their back at the same time, may have spondylolisthesis.

Spondylolisthesis—usually forward slippage of the higher vertebra on the one below it—is described in grades that categorize its severity. Grade I is when the upper vertebra has slipped 25 percent or less across the vertebra below it; grade II is when it has slipped 50 percent; grade III is slippage of 75 percent; and grade IV is more than that. As the slippage progresses, there is usually further narrowing of the neuroforamina. But there is also progressive bending of the spinal cord itself. A garden hose with kinks in it allows the water to trickle rather than flow through it; analogously, with spondylolisthesis, nerve conduction can be severely impaired or, in rare cases, virtually stopped.

Pain from this condition is worse when standing, worse when arching your back, and relieved when you're lying down, especially when curled in the fetal position. This may help distinguish spondylolisthesis from stenosis, but of course spondylolisthesis may be the original cause of the stenosis as well as neuroforaminal narrowing. So what we are really doing here is moving one step back in the chain of causation. Your painful calf is caused, let us say, by pressure on the nerves at L4-L5, which comes from stenosis, which itself may be caused by spondylolisthesis. Because spondylolisthesis can also cause a radiculopathy, your physician will be looking at the neuroforamina too.

It's easy to distinguish this condition from piriformis syndrome, because there are no tender spots; in addition, doing the straight leg test will often make a person who has spondylolisthesis feel better, because the spine curves toward the jutting vertebra, bringing all the vertebrae more into line. But those results are not enough in themselves to make a diagnosis. As usual, the EMG will help figure out which of the nerves are actually affected, but ordinary X-rays will reveal spondylolisthesis every time, and determine its grade. Physical therapy to strengthen abdominal muscles (front, back, and sides), postural training, and a brace* help a vast majority of the time. Myelogram images are generally done before surgery, which is needed perhaps 5 percent of the time.

As of this writing, the National Institute of Arthritis and Musculoskeletal and Skin Diseases is conducting two studies to learn more about the origins of this condition, and to study the role of genes in the progression of the disease. The goal of this research is to identify genetic markers that are associated with differences in the severity of spondylolisthesis and to broaden knowledge about the mechanisms and pathways involved in the development of long-term damage.

SIMPLE MUSCLE SPASM

Sometimes, due to overuse, fatigue, anxiety, pregnancy, electrolyte disorder, or other causes, muscle fibers involuntarily contract and remain in that tightened state for some time. If a muscle in your neck, back, or buttock goes into spasm, you may not be aware that its contraction is the source of your pain.

---

* An abdominal binder with posterior steels and a Velcro closure that can be worn inside a shirt or blouse.

This is the difference between a muscle spasm in your back (or buttock) and a "cramp in your foot," or a "charley horse." Those spasms are extremely painful, and you can feel the muscles clench. Muscle spasms in the back are different. First of all, you can't see them, so you're less aware of their existence and we don't intuitively know what they are. In the case of back muscles, you don't consciously know where they are or when you're using them. Medical schools don't even pay much attention to them.

Also, the muscles in your back aren't like those in your foot or the back of your arm that are responsible for curling your toes or moving your forearm. The muscles in the back have a slightly different function. They are mainly used for support—to keep you upright. Because of this, they're always somewhat contracted. That's normal, and we're used to the contraction and not aware of it. It's difficult to differentiate normal contraction from extreme contraction, which is what happens when one of those muscles goes into spasm.

When it comes to piriformis syndrome, the muscle goes into spasm, but it's not the spasm of the muscle that's painful. It's the muscle squeezing a nerve that's causing the pain.

So you may feel intense pain from almost any back muscle and not know exactly what it's coming from. When muscles go into spasm, they grow shorter, thicker, and stiffer. If a muscle is in chronic spasm, it will become stronger and larger, just like a weight lifter's biceps, and for the same reason.

Nerves that are entrapped in or beneath a contracted muscle—as they can be if muscles near the spine or in the buttocks go into spasm— may be squeezed and cause classic sciatic nerve pain lower down in the body, specifically in the buttocks, legs, and feet. This will go on as long as the muscle is in spasm. If the compression has been intense enough to cause actual nerve damage, it will go on longer. Nerves travel down through the psoas muscle and penetrate or pass closely by many others. We will discuss the anatomy of piriformis syndrome again later.

But, confusingly, many times the muscle itself also hurts. Here's why. When muscles contract, they are working hard and need more blood. There is an irony here, however. Continued contraction compresses the tiny blood vessels (capillaries) that bring in that blood when the muscle needs it most. This shortage of blood during a spasm has three consequences. First, nutrients and oxygen necessary for the muscle's continued contraction are not delivered. Second, waste products of metabolism, such as lactic acid, are not carried away; this leads to irritation of the nerves and muscle fibers and spasm, which cuts down the blood supply still further. The entire cycle goes on and on. But third, reduced oxygen affects the capillaries directly, stimulating them to expand.

Left to its own devices, most spasm will eventually cure itself because of the inherent expansive tendency of oxygen-starved blood vessels to expand. But that often takes time, and during that time you're in pain. However, the inherent elasticity of muscle, which creates the problem, also provides a solution. All you need to do is stretch the muscle, and the blood vessels will enlarge again. The spasm will resolve.

Once in a while, spasm disappears, then quickly returns. If that happens, you can simply stretch the muscle again. Usually 10 to 15 seconds is enough, but sometimes it takes a minute or more. But you have to locate the muscle before you stretch it. And you need to know what the muscle does when it contracts in order to stretch it. The kind of pain caused by a spasm doesn't make the idea of stretching the muscle that hurts very appealing, but it definitely helps. Yoga is an invaluable tool for anyone who is prone to muscle spasm. I discuss at length the yoga poses that can relieve pain and sciatica caused by muscle spasm in my book *Cure Back Pain with Yoga*.

SACROILIAC JOINT DERANGEMENT: WHAT IT IS

This condition is probably the most underdiagnosed and therefore the most undertreated condition that causes lower back pain. It doesn't usually cause sciatica in the strict sense of the word, because it doesn't really involve nerves; it involves joints. It rarely causes pain that goes down the leg; when it does, the pain hardly ever goes lower than the knee. Yet this condition is often associated with another problem—piriformis syndrome—that does cause sciatica. The piriformis muscle inserts at both sides of the sacroiliac joint. When the joint is out of alignment, some but not all of the piriformis muscle fibers are elongated. As a result, the muscle itself may go into spasm. When the piriformis muscle goes into spasm, it may compress the sciatic nerve with enough force to cause sciatica. Sacroiliac (SI) joint derangement is one of the most common causes of piriformis syndrome.

Also, the sacroiliac joint, when deranged or out of alignment, can cause referred pain down the back of the leg that is much like sciatic pain. As already mentioned, that pain rarely, if ever, goes farther than the knee and usually stops much higher up the thigh. Exceptions to this are described in a study that found that leakage of substances from a deranged sacroiliac joint can cause irritation in several ways: by approaching the sciatic nerve from behind and irritating it, by coming close to the lumbosacral plexus in front and causing inflammation there, and by approaching and inflaming the L5-S1 nerve root just above.[35] Sacroiliac joint derangement is different from a radiculopathy and spinal stenosis in that there are no changes in sensation lower down in the body, no numbness, weakness, parasthesias, or bowel or bladder problems, except in the rare circumstances mentioned above. Unlike piriformis syndrome, which is painful with sitting, particularly for long periods, sacroiliac joint derangement is typically worst when you're *rising* from a sitting position (for example, getting out of the seat at the movies), sitting down (in the bathroom), or twisting.

The sacrum is the spade-shaped bone in the center of the back of your pelvis. It's what holds up your entire spinal column and is always considered part of the spinal column itself. This bone looks a little like the cornerstone of a Roman arch and functions the same way. (See illustration on page 90.) Your two legs form the pillars of the arch. The iliac bones form the curved part, and the sacrum is the keystone, the element without which the two sides would collapse. The sacrum is connected to the two iliac bones on the right and the left. These interfaces are the sacroiliac joints.

THE SACRUM moves in three planes: to the right or left, forward or back, or tilted in on the right side or the left. Because it's only one bone, if it's out of kilter on one side—out of joint, or deranged in any of the planes in which it operates—logic dictates that it has to be out of kilter to some extent on the other side. (See illustration on page 91.) For this reason, sacroiliac joint pain frequently (but not always) flickers from right to left and back again.

The sacroiliac joints have complex three-dimensional surfaces, with "stalactites" and "stalagmites" that must fit together perfectly. The joints bear a lot of weight, and the relationship between the bones is central to supporting the myriad, complicated movements of the upper body and the legs. When the sacroiliac joints are functioning properly, you don't even know they're there. But when something is out of kilter, it can hurt like the dickens. This may be because the sacrum stands at the very center of the body. It is the spot where the agile, leveraging, maneuvering upper body and the weight-bearing, supporting lower body interface, and flexibility meets stability. As such, it must adjust to the twist of a golfer's swing, the strain of eight hours sitting in front of a computer screen, and the contortions of lovers. It allows you to hang on to a rail on a bus, carry luggage down the station stairs, and get in to the back seat of a car. If the heart is the core of the circulatory system, the sacrum is the heart of the skeleton.

What causes sacroiliac joint derangement? Stumbles, falls, auto accidents, and other traumas, and lifting and carrying, particularly at awkward angles. Forcible twists are the most common cause of sacroiliac joint derangement. But sometimes there is no identifiable cause at all.

This condition must be diagnosed through a patient's history and a physical exam, not with an EMG or imaging studies. Sacroiliac joint derangement cannot be detected by an EMG because no nerves are directly involved. It's a three-dimensional joint, so most abnormalities cannot be seen on a two-dimensional X-ray or MRI. Your doctor will put his or her thumbs just above and inside your iliac crests (little dimples just above the sacroiliac joint on both sides), then ask you to balance your weight evenly on both feet, and to bend forward. In nine out of ten of the cases of sacroiliac joint derangement that I've seen, one side will

Tensegrity Structure

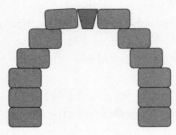

The shape and placement of the sacrum between the hips is exactly the same as that of the keystone of a Roman arch. However, the sacrum also bears a great deal of weight from above, and it mediates between the supportive legs below and the active, twisting, manipulating trunk, arms, and head above.

move appreciably more than the other side, or neither will move much at all. There are other clinical tests, such as Gaenslen's sign, in which holding the entire torso and pelvis still and extending one leg off the edge of an exam table elicits pain in people with SI joint derangement. (See illustration on page 92.)

Many doctors do not accept the possibility that sacroiliac joint derangement exists, and that the sacroiliac joint moves. They believe that the joints don't move at all but become firmly fused at an early age, like the bones of the skull. But although the bony parts of the sacrum itself *do* fuse together, the joints between the whole sacrum and the iliac bones do not. They are a common site of low back pain, and they respond much too well to pain-killing injections and physical therapy to be anything but joints. Yes, I believe firmly that these joints move. Physiatrists, osteopaths, and chiropractors believe that the joints move very slightly, but those few millimeters are crucial to the body functioning painlessly. Because SI joint derangement doesn't show up on imaging tests, physicians and physical therapists rely on physical exam and touch to see whether the joints are symmetrical, and on provoking the pain through

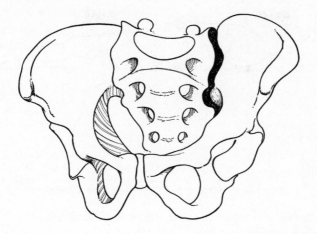

Because the sacrum is one single central bone, it is impossible for it to be out of alignment on one side only. Sacroiliac joint pain therefore frequently vacillates from one side to the other.

movement. Now, however, promising research is being done in the Netherlands on an ultrasound technique that can identify and measure the biomechanical properties of the sacroiliac joint as opposed to that of the pelvic bones,[36] and newer scanning techniques are on the horizon.

I treat sacroiliac joint derangement with nonsteroidal anti-inflammatories to reduce the inflammation, which is almost always there. Sometimes after ten days or so, an injection of steroids into the joint can be helpful in preparing the patient for the definitive treatment—moving the joints back into position. The standard and usually effective physical therapy treatment is based on muscle-energy and strain-counterstrain techniques. I have seen yoga put the joint back into its proper place, and chiropractors are also sometimes successful in doing this.

Once the joint is returned to its original, normal position, it takes about six months before all the sinews around the sacroiliac joint build up the strength and integrity to maintain it as it should be. This is how long connective tissue needs to repair itself; in six months, approximately half the fibers of each ligament holding the joint in place have regrown at the new, proper length, and in the proper position. Those

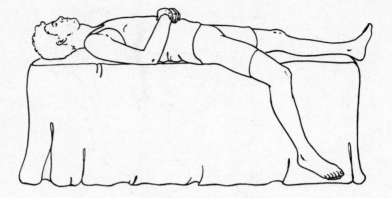

Pain in this position is one of the reasonably reliable tests for sacroiliac joint dysfunction.

strong ligaments are powerful allies when the sacroiliac joint is in place; they're formidable adversaries when it's out of kilter, holding the joint very firmly in the wrong spot. That's why the physical therapist or chiropractor, or whoever treats this problem, has to use a lot of force, often using your leg almost like a crowbar, to push the bones back into place. Once the joint is in proper alignment, I advise you to "walk on eggshells" and refrain from canoeing, vigorous tennis, heavy or repeated lifting, twisting, or any weight workout not done while you lie horizontal on a bench, until the joint is healed.

WHAT YOU CAN DO FOR SACROILIAC JOINT DERANGEMENT AT HOME

The sacroiliac joint usually will repair itself, but it may take months. There are a number of specific exercises that can help it along. One, in particular, I call "leaning" (see page 111 and illustration on page 112), which appears in my previous book *Back Pain: How to Diagnose and Cure Low Back Pain and Sciatica.* Once I used this exercise to cure a young man of sacroiliac joint derangement over the phone. I was explaining to him how he could put two chairs back-to-back and just far enough apart so he could fit between them. He was to put his hands on the backs of the chairs, and support most of his weight on his arms. His legs would come close to dangling, allowing gravity to slip his sacroiliac joint back into place. He couldn't do what I was instructing and hold the phone at the same time, so he put down the receiver. A moment later I heard a lot of laughter from the other end, and shouts of what I can only describe as happiness.

OSTEOARTHRITIS: WHAT IT IS

Osteoarthritis is a process that is almost inevitable in anyone over the age of eighteen. Joints in the human body are moving structures, of course, but they're not alive in the conventional sense of the word. The cartilage and elastic tissue that make up the inner linings of the joints— the parts of any two bones that come closest to each other throughout the body—are not alive. Like hair, like fingernails and toenails, like tears, these materials are continuously secreted by live tissue but are not themselves made up of live cells. Because they're not alive, you wouldn't expect that age would change them. Time, however, does make a difference, because the cells in the cartilage and beneath joint linings do get older and do change.

If you dissected a joint, you would see two inside surfaces, with every nook and cranny, every bend and bay mirrored by the opposite surface. The ball of the joint at the femur fits precisely into the hollow socket of the hip. They are concentric spheres. They grow this way under instructions from your genetic code; but as years go by, natural wear and tear is hard on the cartilage. That's not so serious, though, because that material is being replaced on a continuous basis, just like hair or nails. Less happily, the orientation of the cells below, which are producing the cartilage, also begins to change. If the cells that produce cartilage for the head of the femur, let's say, are no longer as efficient or smooth as they once were, that will affect not only the head of the femur; it will concentrate pressure on the opposite surface—the socket in the pelvis. That socket will be changed slowly, which will reflect back and further alter the ball of the femur, and so on. This vicious cycle is the main process of osteoarthritis.

But problems with the underlying manufacture of cartilage in the joints of the spine as well as elsewhere are not the only cause of this disease. You can suffer damage because of a bacterial infection in the joint; you can experience trauma; or you can hurt the surfaces of the inside of the joint by moving repetitively in an unusual way. Autoimmune diseases such as rheumatoid arthritis attack the joints, as can Lyme disease. A similar phenomenon occurs at the ends of bone, just inside their joint capsules (envelopes of protective tissue) and cartilage. Instead of the smooth, neat edges that characterize the healthy bones of a 20-year-old, irregularities, growths, and erosions appear on the bone's surface near the joint cartilage. But the underlying mechanism is always the same: malformations in underlying tissue produce surfaces that no longer fit together perfectly.

What can you do? Osteoarthritis strikes every animal that has joints. It thickens the bones, narrows the joints, and inflames the membranes that enclose them. As bones get thicker, the openings in them become narrower. When this narrowing is in the spine, it may cause radiculopathy or stenosis. The situation is then complicated by inflammation, which is inherent in rheumatoid arthritis and seems to be brought about by the degenerative changes in osteoarthritis. Nonsteroidal anti-inflammatories can be useful.

When there is stenosis or radiculopathy, steroids are an option, as are procedures such as radio frequency ablation to relieve painful nerve entrapments and surgery to reshape irregular cartilage and remove impinging bone. Physical therapy and yoga can be helpful for increasing range of motion. If you get 3 degrees of extra motion at every vertebra, that's 90 degrees of added motion for the spine.

OSTEOPOROSIS

Most people who have osteoporosis are women over the age of sixty, but this degenerative condition can also affect men. Osteoporosis is a cause of back pain, but not of sciatica.

Whereas joints may not be alive, bones are; and like many other parts of our body, cells inside them are constantly dying and regenerating. Constituent tissue, consisting of a protein matrix and minerals such as calcium and phosphates, goes through a complete life cycle and is totally replaced every seven years or so. Two kinds of cells are responsible for this replacement process. The first are osteocytes, which lay down the protein matrix, called osteoid, by taking protein elements out of the blood and synthesizing long molecules. The osteoid then draws calcium and phosphate into it, thereby hardening into bone. The second kind of cells, osteoclasts, are large cells with many nuclei; they return the mineral elements to the bloodstream to regulate the body's level of circulating calcium and phosphate, for later redeposit in the bones or for excretion. Balancing the activity of these two kinds of cells is a complex task involving hormones, exercise, sunlight, and many other factors. In other words, the backbone's connected to the bloodstream.

Bones contain 99 percent of all the body's calcium, and that is where we get calcium when we need it. Muscles function properly in a narrow range of calcium concentration. If the calcium concentration gets too high or too low, the result can be painful tightening of the muscles and life-threatening spasm of the muscles and the heart. Therefore the body keeps very close tabs on calcium, taking it relentlessly from the bones whenever needed. Chemical signals are transmitted to the osteoclasts by the bloodstream to regulate this process.

Younger people secrete more osteoid than they reabsorb, and thereby grow. Mature individuals have virtually equal activities of creation and reabsorption, although many older people find themselves in the reverse position: they are losing more bone substance than their osteocytes are generating.

This pathological condition occurs when new bone formation and old bone reabsorption are not in balance. Insufficient calcium and vitamin D intake are contributing factors; so are smoking, lack of exercise, and some eating disorders. A lack of estrogen in women and androgen in men is also associated with bone loss, which occurs over a period of many years.

Osteoporosis is characterized by weaker, less dense bones, which are fragile and prone to breaking. Those places where fractures are most likely are in the hip, thoracic and lumbar spine, and wrist. Spinal or vertebral fractures can have serious consequences, including severe back pain, loss of height, and deformity. Occasionally these fractures are unstable, causing nerve damage.

Treatments for fractures include bracing and arthroscopic "gluing" with epoxy. Postural changes often provide good relief. But the best treatment is prevention. Excellent medicines such as Actonel, Fosamax, and Evista are available, and exercise such as yoga has shown promise as a means of stimulating the mechanoreceptors in osteocytes that prompt them to produce more bone.

FACET SYNDROME: WHAT IT IS

This is a problem with the small joints that connect the vertebrae to one another. Each vertebra has two of these joints going to the vertebra above it and two going to the vertebra below. These joints are miniatures of bigger joints in other places in the body and have all the same structures: joint linings, synovial fluid, capsules, elastin, and collagen.

Like bigger joints, facet joints can get into trouble for a variety of reasons. When they do—whether the joints have simply slipped by one another, producing great pain; or osteoarthritis has caused irregularities in their surfaces; or an individual has had an accident or fall—the joints can cause radiating pain that is easily confused with sciatic pain. The difference between that pain and the pain of sciatica is that there is no numbness, weakness, or bowel or bladder involvement, and only rarely strange sensations.

Facet syndrome rarely occurs on both sides or at more than one spinal level at any one time. Neither sitting nor standing relieves the pain. This condition is not nearly as common as was once thought. In the past, stiff muscles that were causing pain and reducing range of motion in a small section of the spine were often diagnosed as facet syndrome. A more appropriate term for this has appeared in recent literature—"segmental rigidity" (see below).

A recent study showed that 72.1 percent of patients given facet injections of steroid, Lidocaine, and iopamidol under fluoroscopic guidance had a good response after 3 weeks. Although this number dropped to 31.4 percent after 12 weeks, it was far superior to what was seen in a control group.[37] These were patients with normal MRIs, no signs of nerve root involvement, and no history of back pain. A more recent study randomized patients who were diagnosed with the recently identified condition called "segmental rigidity"[38]; it can follow back surgery or come at other times when people have firm and relatively immobile segments of their spine, generally in the lower lumbar region. Patients were randomized, and injections were given to those with spinal segmental rigidity and those without it. After the injections, the patients were evaluated for "facet syndrome." Surprisingly, it turned out that only 15 to 19 percent of the patients in each group had facet syndrome, and the injection seemed to work well for those in both groups. All of these patients also received stretching exercises and physical therapy. So these injections work well to stretch out rigidity in spinal segments whether or not there is facet syndrome. It appears that the injection relaxes painfully tight muscles near the joint.

In 2004 researchers at the University of Texas, examining 421 patients over a period of time, found that they could independently identify and estimate the severity of segmental rigidity. In this group only 17 percent of the patients actually had facet syndrome.[39] Nevertheless, facet injections and exercise helped up to 97 percent of the patients improve their range of motion. A much lower percentage of patients in an exercise-only control group improved.

Our choice of treatment for this problem, once it is diagnosed by a physician's exam and X-ray, is physical therapy. A radiographically guided injection of steroids and local anesthetic into the facet joint can be used as a diagnostic tool as well as a therapeutic procedure, according to a study published in *Clinical Orthopaedics*.[40]

INFECTION AND SCIATICA

Does your back suddenly hurt like crazy? Do you have other viral or flu-like symptoms, such as fever or cough? Are your eyes unusually sensitive to light? If you have the last symptom and a stiff neck—so you are unable to bring your chin down to your chest with your mouth closed—go to an emergency room. Meningitis, which has viral and bacterial forms, can cause pain and can be serious. A test of your spinal fluid, done in the hospital, can determine in less than an hour whether you have meningitis.

TUMORS

Occasionally tumors occur in the spinal column. Whether a tumor is benign or malignant, it can take up space. A malignant spinal tumor is usually a metastasis from another location—the lung, colon, prostate, breast, ovary, or kidney. I've taken care of patients whose first symptom was back pain and they turned out to have a serious form of cancer, but that is an extremely rare situation; in a quarter of a century I've seen this only twice. Benign tumors such as meningiomas and tarlov cysts are more common, but they rarely cause pain or sciatica unless they press against spinal rootlets, which does happen occasionally. Tumors are best diagnosed with a CT scan or MRI, then treated with scalpel or gamma knife. Use of the gamma knife is also known as radiosurgery—a technique using highly focused beams of cobalt 60 radiation instead of a conventional incision.

Rarely, there can be a problem in the lumbosacral plexus at the sides of the bottom of the spine. A baby's head rests near there on its way to the birth canal and can put pressure on parts of the nerve-containing plexus. Colon or ovarian cancer can also spread into that area. In this type of situation, pelvic symptoms, bladder and bowel changes, and intestinal upsets could occur along with sciatica, although I have seen this only once.

MULTIPLE SCLEROSIS AND STROKE

These conditions of the central nervous system sometimes cause pain in the sciatic distribution by affecting nerve fibers or nuclei anywhere in the spine, the neck, or even the brain. Treatment recommendations are beyond the scope of this book, but see my book *Yoga in the Treatment of Multiple Sclerosis and Neurological Conditions*, published by Demos Press in August 2006. There I have included a physical therapeutic approach with demonstrable results.

Part II

CONTROL and CURE

Chapter VI

OUTSMART SCIATICA WITH TRICKS YOU CAN DO ON YOUR OWN

STRENGTHEN YOUR ABS, TORSO, AND CORE. A six-pack may not be in your future, but let's face it: muscles hold your body together, and they hold it up. The weaker your abdominal muscles, the more likely you are to have problems with your back. Ironically, strengthening one set of abdominal muscles while ignoring another may actually cause or worsen back pain, not relieve it. To avoid this situation, I recommend that you educate yourself about Pilates, yoga, Alexander technique, Feldenkrais method, and/or old-fashioned calisthenics. Always do exercises of any type symmetrically. In other words, if you do something involving your right arm or leg, make sure you do the same thing with the left arm or leg as well. The exception is with scoliosis, which is rarely painful and is beyond the scope of the discussion here.

You can get exercise videos, read books, go to the gym, or take classes. But do exercise. Think about how many times you've said to yourself or heard a friend say, "As long as I exercise regularly, I can keep my back in pretty good shape." Swimming is also helpful for general strengthening.

Many of my patients, especially those who are overweight, tell me they don't have time to exercise, aren't motivated, or it's too painful. My answer to that is: if you want to prevent back pain, you must have some self-discipline. Become motivated, set goals, exercise every day or every other day, and begin a habit you won't want to break.

For specific abdominal strengthening exercises, you can visit the Web sites of the American Academy of Orthopaedic Surgeons, the Georgia State University Department of Kinesiology and Health, and the Mayo Clinic. Try the exercises you find there to the best of your ability, neither overdoing it nor slacking off. Whether or not you have a six-pack, make strengthening a habit, and you will look and feel better.

CHANGE IFFY ROUTINES. Have you been wearing the same shoes almost every day for the past month? Watching television all evening curled in the same favorite but lumpy chair? Have you carried the same briefcase, and in the same hand, for the past year? If you have, join the club. We're all extremely loyal to our habits—even the bad ones.

A backache often heralds a siege of sciatica. Also, backaches are often caused by something you're doing, such as the way you sit in bed each night and read before you fall asleep. If your back begins to ache, it's well worth becoming alert to your own movements and patterns and carefully observing your physical reactions. No one is better equipped than you are to link your behaviors with the twinges they cause in your back. When you discover a possible cause of back pain, be bold. Switch shoes, switch the shoulder on which you usually carry your handbag, or stop carrying a handbag at all for a couple of weeks. Stop the repetitive activity you've been doing (even if it's exercise); move the car seat position, or get someone else to do the driving and sit in back.

If you have back pain and spend many hours a day at a computer workstation, make sure that your environment is set up to keep your back healthy, using ergonomics. This science includes equipment design, often for the workplace. Ergonomically designed environments are intended to maximize productivity by reducing fatigue, discomfort, and injury. Ergonomics overlaps biotechnology, human engineering, and human factors engineering. Specialists in these fields pay attention to a whole range of things that most of us may not even think about, such as the height of the call button on the elevator, or what it takes to dismantle the toaster oven for cleaning, or the correct angle for the car seat back to minimize back fatigue. Many large companies employ ergonomic specialists to keep employees productive. If you don't work for one of those companies, look in the telephone book to find ergonomic specialists who will analyze your workstation or your home. Or you can get online advice from the U.S. Department of Labor, Occupational Safety and Health Administration,[41] if your computer desk is not set up to keep your back healthy, or you need to change the position of your car seat when you commute to and from work.

EXERCISE ROUTINE A BACK PAIN SUSPECT? If you think it's the yoga, the six-mile jogs, or lifting those weights, just stop everything for three or four days. When the pain subsides, add exercises back into your routine one by one, just the way you would add foods to the diet of a child who appears to have allergies. If you're sure that your exercises are causing pain, see a specialist in physical medicine and rehabilitation to develop a program that is likely to help, not hurt. Obviously, consult a medical professional if you're not sure what's causing pain that goes on for more than two weeks.

COMMIT TO CORRECT POSTURE. Poor posture is frequently related to back pain, as is a problem with the way you walk—a gait abnormality or irregularity. In short, try to stay aware of your posture and stand upright. Yoga is particularly effective for helping you do this. See the pose called Tadasana, or Standing Mountain, in my previous book *Cure Back Pain with Yoga*. Good posture means that your head, neck, torso, buttocks, and legs are aligned. Not one section of your body should slump. Good posture should also apply to the way you sit, walk, and sleep. If you suspect that you have a gait abnormality, have the way you walk evaluated by a physical therapist or other professional so that any problem can be corrected.

Leg length discrepancies of less than a quarter of an inch are almost expected in most individuals. Sometimes, because of fractures, illnesses, or other factors, there are bigger differences. In that case a simple in-shoe lift may do a good deal to relieve lower back pain. Wear a quarter-inch lift for an hour or so the first day, then wear it a little longer until after two weeks you're wearing it all the time. The lift should be made of cork, leather, or plastic, not the "soft" gel that will be squashed to almost nothing when you put your weight on it.

STRETCH. As I've said many times, vigorous exercise is often curative where back pain is concerned. Exercise will warm you up and get your heart beating strongly. Stretching, the antidote to fatigue, is just as important as exercise for separating tight structures and easing pain. Many of the modalities (yoga, Pilates, Feldenkrais) discussed in these pages provide a structured way to stretch, reducing spasm, helping to solve postural problems, and cutting down on the physical correlates of stress. If your work necessitates repetitive movements, stretching can counteract their negative effects. Lengthening your muscles, strengthening them, and keeping them limber is a general way to cope with, cure, and prevent sciatica.

LIFT CORRECTLY. It's the groceries, the suitcase, the box full of old books. It's the bricks you're using to edge the lawn, the computer component, the spilled peanuts under the heavy living room easy chair, the chubby toddler who wants up. Not lifting correctly (especially if you twist a little at the same time) can get you into big trouble. If you've already got a backache, it's madness to lift even a mildly heavy object incorrectly.

When lifting, remember that your back should not be doing the hard work. Leave that labor for the powerful muscles in the buttocks and the thighs. Give yourself a solid foundation when you have to lift something heavy by always bending your knees. Keep your trunk vertical. If you lean over so that your trunk is horizontal, you're creating leverage that adds hundreds or thousands of extra pounds of pressure to the structures of your lower back. Leaning over while lifting endangers your disks, strains your muscles, and overstretches your ligaments and all the elements of your vertebral and sacroiliac joints.

One cardinal rule of proper lifting: get close to the object, whether you're lifting it from the floor, bringing it down from a shelf, or accepting it from another person. If someone is handing you a heavy object, bend your knees, keep your back straight, and get as near to the object as possible so you can receive it at waist height if possible.

RELAX. It sounds nice, it is nice, and it does help.[42] When you relax, those tight muscles pulling and pinching loosen up. You have the opportunity to change your focus to something other than pain. Tight muscles are not just a physiological phenomenon; they have a psychological component too. Calming down enough to gain mental access to the part of your brain that controls the tight muscles is an effective means of dealing with pain. The longer the pain drags on, the more it drags you down. Relaxation is a reprieve. I recommend it as a preventative as well as for relief.

CHAIR TRICKS

BENDS. Try this if you have stenosis, spondylolisthesis, piriformis syndrome, herniated disk, or arthritis. Sit comfortably in a straight wooden chair. Your feet are on the floor, forearms on your thighs, and palms on your knees. Gradually slide your forearms forward. Your feet remain flat on the floor. Keep your spine straight. Your arms, not your back, should be holding you up, bearing your weight. Leaning forward stretches the muscles of your buttocks and lower back without stretching the nerves. It does, however, move the sciatic nerve a tiny bit, opening the neuroforamina through which spinal nerve roots pass. It eases the pressure on the sacroiliac joint. Try this simple exercise when you're in pain and feeling bad.

TWISTS. This particular twist is good for arthritis, sacroiliac joint derangement, piriformis syndrome, and stenosis. It's not good for herniated disk or spondylolisthesis. If it hurts, stop. Sit toward the front of the seat of an armchair, feet flat on the floor, knees together and pointing

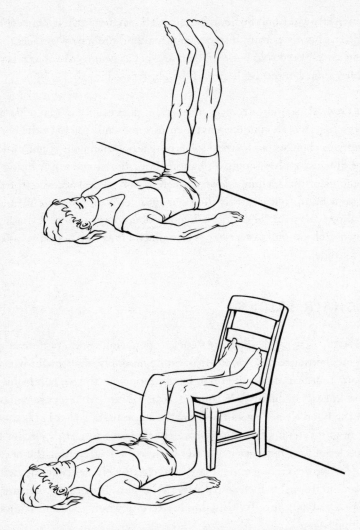

This position is excellent for spondylolisthesis, spinal stenosis, and many cases of piriformis syndrome. Use the chair version at first, especially in cases of significant hypertension, congestive heart failure, or glaucoma. People with cerebrovascular compromise or the threat of it must avoid this position entirely.

straight ahead. Bring your right hand over to the left chair arm. Your left hand reaches behind you toward the right chair arm or all the way to it. Let your right chest move forward and your left arm pull your left shoulder back. Sit up straight.

Another chair twist involves straddling an armless chair. Your right hand goes to the left side of the chair back. Your left hand goes behind you to the right side of the seat. Twist your torso, keeping it upright, with your right chest and arm moving forward and to the left at the same time. This is good for arthritis, sacroiliac joint derangement, piriformis syndrome, and stenosis. Don't do this exercise if you have herniated disk or spondylolisthesis.

WALL TRICKS

LEGS UP. If you have a pinched nerve or pinched nerves because of stenosis, this exercise—which reduces the constriction of nerve openings—is one of the most comforting things you can do for yourself. Lie on the floor with your buttocks close to a wall. Put your legs straight up against the wall parallel to each other. (See illustration on page 108.) Let them rest there for as long as you want. To come down, bend one knee, roll to that side, and bring that leg and foot to the floor. Repeat this exercise as often as you like. You can lie on soft cushions to do it. If you cannot straighten your knees against the wall, you can do a modified version of this exercise by lying on the floor and resting your calves on the seat of an upholstered chair (see illustration). This relaxes the lower back muscles and buttock muscles, stretches the bony covering of the spinal cord, and thins the nerves, reducing compression in the spine and at the piriformis muscle. People with cerebrovascular disease, wet macular degeneration, or congestive heart failure should consult their physicians before attempting these positions.

WALL DOG. This variation of a yoga pose called Upward Facing Dog increases the range of motion of the entire spine and coordinates the muscles that move it. It also stretches the back of the hip joint, a prob-

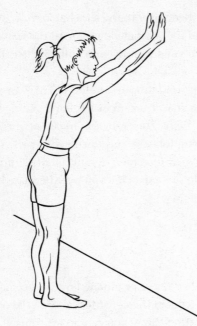

This pose extends the thoracic spine, improving posture and moving the spinal cord within the bony canal of the vertebral column. It may relieve acute or chronic pain due to narrowing of the lumbar canal, adhesions, or kyphosis, and sometimes nerve roots pinched by herniated lumbar disks.

lem area for many people who have piriformis syndrome. Here's how to do it (see illustration on page 110). Stand about a foot away from a wall and facing it. Pay attention to your posture. Distribute your weight evenly on your feet, and look straight ahead. Now place your palms high on the wall, well above eye level and a few inches wider apart than your shoulders. Your fingers should point up. Keeping your knees and elbows straight, pull your hips back, and bring your armpits forward and as close to the wall as possible (see illustration). It's easy to arch your lower back, but in this pose you must do something more difficult: arch your upper back by bringing your sternum toward the wall. Keep your elbows straight. Your forehead will move toward the wall but should not touch it. This is good for sacroiliac joint derangement, herniated disk, musculoskeletal pain, piriformis syndrome, and segmental rigidity. Do not do this if you have spondylolisthesis.

STANDING TRICKS

LEANING. This exercise stretches the muscles between the pelvis and thoracic spine and helps with sacroiliac joint derangement, spondylolisthesis, segmental rigidity, and herniated disk. Because the sacroiliac joint is such a significant factor in piriformis syndrome, this exercise helps piriformis syndrome too. Do it for short periods of time, so the muscles don't contract.

Stand facing and close to a kitchen counter, table, or any other stable object about waist height. Your feet should be comfortably apart. With your palms facing away from your body, lean forward slowly, digging your elbows into your lower ribs, until the heels of your hands come to rest on the edge of the counter. (See illustration on page 112.) Your forearms should support most but not all of your weight. Your feet and legs should do little weight bearing, and your heels will lift slightly off the floor. It's very important to relax your abdominal muscles. You are doing this exercise correctly when you feel a stretch—and a dull or not so dull pain—in your lower back. Lean like this for up to 20 seconds as many times a day as you like; as it becomes comfortable, increase the time.

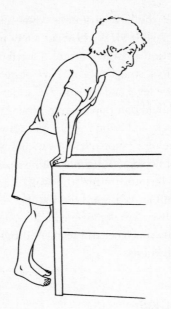

Pressing the elbows into the lower ribs and leaning forward lifts the spinal cord just slightly, while gravity pulls the hips and pelvis down, allowing the sacroiliac joint to equilibrate.

BARFLIES' TRICK. Did you ever notice that the regulars in the corner bar stand for long hours, nursing their drinks, listening to the jukebox, talking to their companions or the bartender? Maybe you weren't aware of the feet of those regulars, who are as prone to backache as everyone else. While they stand there sipping their beers, or even when they're sitting on a bar stool to imbibe, they tend to rest one foot on the low rail that runs the length of the bar at ankle height. You may not be a regular at any bar, but you can learn something important from those who are. Employ their trick when you're standing and when you're sitting, no matter where you are. If you can perch one foot even six inches off the floor by resting it on a ledge, the bottom step of a staircase, a chair rail, even a telephone book, you will find that it relieves pain. It relaxes the muscles of the lower spine and relieves constriction at nerve openings. This is good for all back conditions, except possibly compression fracture.

CLOTHING TRICKS

LIGHTEN YOUR LOAD. If you're like me and my wife, you've been carrying your purse or briefcase on a shoulder strap for years, almost wearing a groove into your skin and bone. This asymmetrical weight is bad for anyone with sciatica. A backpack, which at least distributes the weight evenly on both sides of your body, is an improvement. Another solution is to have duplicate sets of things that you keep in different locations, so you take with you only what you need. You can have a makeup kit at home and in the office, for example, keeping the cosmetics in your purse to a minimum. By the same token, you might be lugging certain papers back and forth from the office to your home but not looking at them at all. If you must carry a heavy load on one shoulder or in one hand, be fair to your back: change shoulders or sides frequently to distribute the work more evenly.

WEAR THE RIGHT SHOES, AND USE ORTHOTICS. If the shoe doesn't fit, don't wear it. Shoes are famous culprits in back pain and sciatica. If you have back pain, you can ignore Lord Chesterton's famous advice to "Eat to please yourself; dress to please others." You should wear shoes that please your feet.

Shoes need to do more than fit; they must also cushion the feet and allow them to do their job properly. Shoes are, of course, the actual foundation of our balance when we are standing up. They influence posture just as leg and foot abnormalities do. Flat shoes encourage the wearer to tilt the top of the pelvis back, decreasing the arch of the back and tucking in the buttocks. Flat shoes help if you have piriformis syndrome.

High heels—and they are higher now than ever before in my memory—throw the body's weight forward, giving the back more arch and the pelvis more motion in walking. This is good for those who have herniated disk and don't have sacroiliac joint derangement, but may be particularly hazardous for anyone who has spondylolisthesis or spinal stenosis.

Then there are the narrow, pointed shoe beds. Even if the foot sits far back from that pointy toe, squeezing it into a narrow space isn't beneficial. Also, when there is a lot of empty (pointed) shoe in front of your toes, you're more likely to trip and fall. Such an imbalance tightens abdominal and back muscles in an unfortunate opposition to one another. For anyone with a pinched nerve, the feeling in the feet or toes may already be compromised, so you may not be aware that you are causing injury to the foot. Whether or not your shoes are hurting or compromising your feet, it's a good idea to change them frequently. Some people change their shoes every day; others change them several times a day.

If you have problems with your gait or posture that are making your back pain and sciatica worse, shoe inserts or orthotics may bring you a great deal of relief. A doctor of physical medicine and rehabilitation, a neurologist, an orthopedist, or a podiatrist can prescribe inserts to correct your particular problem.

WEAR AN ABDOMINAL BINDER. For disk problems, spondylolisthesis, or arthritis, wearing an abdominal binder with "steels" in the back for a few weeks can provide support and comfort. The steels are actually slat-like pieces of plastic, wood, or steel that slide into the back of the brace to give it strength without appreciably increasing its weight. Just as important as support, the brace can help make you more aware of your posture and promote its improvement. The brace keeps the body more aligned and takes some strain off muscles while getting the bones to do more of the work. Abdominal binders come in many widths, with special adaptations for patients who have spondylolisthesis and vertebral fractures. Wearing a binder does, however, reduce muscle use, so you should have a consistent exercise program to maintain and increase your strength. Eventually stronger torso muscles supplant the function of the binder, and you can then stow it in the closet.

BED TRICKS

CURL UP. The fetal position is ideal for someone who has a backache or sciatica. It relieves the pain of herniated disk, sacroiliac joint derangement, spondylolisthesis, piriformis syndrome, and arthritis. Lie comfortably on one side, and bring your knees up toward your chest. A pillow placed between your legs can reduce the pressure on your lower hip and the weight of your legs pulling on one side of your spine. As long as you don't curl up so tightly that you aggravate your pain, you can stay in this position as long as you like.

ACQUIRE PILLOWS AND CUSHIONS. Pillows and cushions come in all shapes, sizes, and density. Use them with imagination. Stuff one under your hip, place one at the back of your neck, let your knees rest on a long bolster. There is no right or wrong way to use pillows. Although I'm suggesting here that you use them liberally while lying in bed, you can also use them while sitting in a chair, sitting in bed, lying on a couch, or even when resting on the floor.

SOAK IN A WARM TUB. Submerge yourself to the chin in a tub full of warm (not too hot) water and let it soothe the pain of sciatica, sacroiliac joint derangement, and piriformis syndrome. The buoyancy of the water counteracts the force of gravity, and the warmth is relaxing. I know people who follow every visit to the gym or health club with a warm bath to help prevent old injuries from flaring up and to relax after a workout. You should probably not soak more than twenty minutes once a day, three times a week, although you can add bath oil to avoid drying out your skin. You're not in bed, but you are lying down.

Chapter VII

PHYSICAL
THERAPY

PHYSICAL THERAPY IS ONE of the first standard treatments prescribed by doctors for low back pain or sciatica. This conservative treatment, in addition to nonsteroidal anti-inflammatories, is intended to reduce spasticity, help restore function, improve mobility, relieve pain, and prevent further episodes. In addition, physical therapy aims to restore, maintain, and encourage overall fitness and health. Your physical therapist (PT) should be licensed by the state and have an advanced degree and supervised clinical experience. He or she will educate you about your condition or diagnosis and help you with exercise, using various manual techniques and treatment augmented by heat, cold, ultrasound, or several forms of electricity. All this is designed to facilitate healing and prevent reinjury.

Like doctors, physical therapists frequently specialize. Low back pain patients benefit from therapists who have an orthopedic orientation and education in the treatment of neurological conditions that can be relieved by exercises to restore motor function and improve range of motion. PTs are also qualified to analyze you in relation to your environment and address issues such as chair height and the necessity for shoe inserts.

In some states you need a doctor's prescription to see a physical therapist. In other states you can go to a physical therapist without a doctor's order. Whether or not the laws allow direct access without having seen a doctor, the therapist is trained to assess your condition with a thorough physical exam. The therapist looks for red flags warning that you need a referral to a doctor for a problem that can't be treated by physical therapy and perhaps is potentially serious. Therapists are able to refer you to the proper doctor if necessary.

Even if your doctor has sent you for physical therapy, you may not have an official diagnosis or precise physical therapy recommendations. Your doctor may simply write on the prescription, "Low back pain. Evaluate and treat." This is because sometimes the diagnosis alone is not as important as the physical therapist assessing your body's movement patterns to see where the problem lies. For instance, is it weakness or muscle imbalance that is limiting your movement and aggravating your pain?

The therapist you see may be in the physician's office or in an independent setting. Having seen or not seen your medical records, the therapist will assess your condition and embark on a treatment plan.

If your primary care physician sends you to a chiropractor, podiatrist, osteopath, physiatrist, or surgeon, treatments are distinct and more or less predictable. With physical therapy, it's not quite as straightforward. You go to the therapist, and that person may take over your care, at times without direct communication with your physician. Physical therapy includes a large range of treatments, and your therapist may have particular strengths and approaches, and concentrate more on one type of therapy than another. Because of that, if you are sent to two different therapists, you might receive two different treatments; the only way you'll know if you're receiving the right care is if your pain subsides. I recommend discussing your diagnosis (or lack of it) with your doctor and your physical therapist, to get as much information as possible about your condition and the treatment you are receiving.

An important factor in the success of physical therapy is frequency. A cousin of mine once had a severe backache, and I recommended physical therapy. She went to two sessions but couldn't fit regular visits into her busy work schedule. Finally the therapist said, "You're not a good patient." My cousin was shocked. "I thought I was doing everything you told me to do," she replied. "Yes," said the therapist, "but that was for a hundred and five minutes in the month of May. Now it's July." I would advise any patient receiving physical therapy to put everything else aside and go as often as you're told until the PT says it's no longer necessary, and your improvement confirms that. Going sporadically or quitting before you have significant improvement may help a little, but you can't assume that healing will continue or even persist without regular sessions.

Another factor especially critical for treating back pain and sciatica is doing the therapeutic exercises and home routines the therapist advises, not only while you're being treated but after you have completed direct treatment. Home exercise programs are key to decreasing pain between therapy appointments and absolutely essential for achieving, then main-taining, a pain-free condition.

Once you are discharged from therapy, you will almost certainly be given a program of home exercises, which you may be able to discon-tinue after a while. If your pain should flare up—in a week or in three months—you should try doing these exercises and treating yourself. These regimens are also a means of preventing re-injury. They are signif-icant in that they are tailored for your body by someone who knows you and is familiar with your problem. No other practitioner can readily give you these.

Back pain and sciatica patients benefit from exercises that focus on lumbo-pelvic, or core, stabilization, according to Stephanie Leaf, a phys-ical therapist practicing in New York City. These exercises usually involve strengthening muscles of the abdomen and torso, or pelvic tilts, but of course specific exercises are always tailored to the particular patient. Pilates exercises are useful for developing core strength.

PHYSICAL THERAPY MODALITIES

HEAT AND COLD. The use of heat is well known and has even been successful on a long-term basis, for example, to relieve pain and reduce muscle stiffness and disability while patients are sleeping at night.

Heat induces blood vessels to dilate just below the skin, but that placement actually serves to reduce the effectiveness of the heat. Dilated blood vessels carry heat away the same way a car radiator does, so the warmth never gets more than a few millimeters below the skin's surface. Still, heat does help you relax, and that prepares you for physical mobilizations of other kinds.[43]

Cold is usually applied with ice or sprays. The cooling is anesthetic, which heat is not. Cold makes blood vessels constrict; therefore, it penetrates much more deeply than heat. Although cold has no relaxing properties, it does reduce swelling and slow down the chemical reactions that mediate inflammation and pain. It may be used after an aggressive therapy session to reduce tenderness and inflammation; it may prevent inflammation occurring with injury; and it may aid the healing process. Nevertheless, cold isn't used as often as heat in physical therapy.

ELECTRICITY APPLIED TO MUSCLES. Of course many clinical devices are powered by electricity, but physical therapy also uses electricity directly in many ways that bring a great deal of relief. Electrical stimulation makes muscles contract therapeutically. Different waveforms and amplitudes are used to tire out muscle fibers (which reduces spasm and muscle tightness) or to aid in muscle contraction (which helps correct muscle weakness or imbalance for certain actions, such as walking). This technique is called functional electrical stimulation, or FES. It may involve a portable stimulating activator that goes into action, for example, when a patient's heel strikes the floor. It has not yet become as successful as initially hoped, but this may be due to underestimating the complexity of human neural equipment. Still, many types of electricity can provide pain relief and aid the therapist in facilitating mobilization.

TENS (TRANSCUTANEOUS NERVE STIMULATION). This application of electricity directly to nerves is used in the acute state of an injury to decrease pain and allow for the use of passive, active assisted, or active movement that will begin to correct the disorder. For chronic problems, TENS keeps pain fibers occupied with the use of innocuous stimuli, blocking the reception of impulses that relay actual pain so that an individual gains a sense of well-being and loses nothing.

This is what happens: electrodes are attached between the small TENS machine and the skin near pain sites. Then a mild electrical current is administered, sometimes in pulses, and sometimes in conjunction with heat. This current is strong enough to be felt but not intense enough to excite pain receptors. The feeling that patients describe when TENS is being administered is buzzing or tingling. The idea is that your brain has a limited number of pain receptors, and the electrical current sent into your body occupies so many of them in a harmless way that there aren't enough left to register much pain. TENS acts like a gate at the brain's pain centers, to close or block off pain, though often the relief is transient, and of course any relief is symptomatic and doesn't correct the original problem. However, many injuries and much pain is self-correcting and short-lived, so occupying the receptor sites for a week or so may be enough to outlast the problem.

The theory behind this therapy was developed by pain research giants Ronald Melzack and Patrick Wall. Many of my patients tell me that TENS is helpful, but the medical literature on this subject is inconclusive. There are no harmful side effects to this treatment.

ELECTRICAL STIMULATION (ES). Electrical interference can stimulate some muscle fibers to contract, taking control away from the patient. After a time, that muscle, stimulated externally, tires out and relaxes from sheer fatigue. Spasm disappears. Low or high voltage can be used in the same way to get rid of muscle spasm.

ULTRASOUND. High-frequency sound waves are generated and used to treat various injuries via an instrument that looks something like a telephone receiver. The sound waves travel deep into the affected area, creating gentle, penetrating heat to help relax tight muscles and reduce the pain of spasm. Ultrasound is sometimes administered as a sort of massage, using steroid cream as a lubricant, which helps reduce inflammation. This treatment also promotes circulation, and therefore healing.

MECHANICAL TECHNIQUES

Movement should never be underestimated as a means of relieving lower back pain. Mechanical and movement techniques used in physical therapy are so diverse that they're hard to characterize. They include manual mobilizations of affected areas to help you stretch and increase mobility and flexibility, and exercises that you do yourself. Manual therapeutic techniques often used for back pain and sciatica include joint mobilizations, muscle energy, strain-counterstrain, myofascial release, passive stretching, and other hands-on techniques performed by you and your physical therapist.

ACTIVE ASSISTED RANGE OF MOTION. The therapist helps you lift and move for gentle stretching and strengthening. This is done to augment specific limited movement ranges of joints and muscles.

EXTENSION AND FLEXION BACK EXERCISES. These exercises improve muscle tone and strength, relieve pain, and prevent recurrence of injury. They may help move a bulging disk into a more normal place, then strengthen surrounding musculature to prevent another occurrence of "slipped" disk.

ISOMETRIC EXERCISE. Contracting muscles without moving, to increase strength.

ISOTONIC EXERCISE. A constant resistance to motion in specific range of motion exercises, to increase strength.

JOINT MOBILIZATION. The therapist stretches the joint until it reaches its limit, then helps it go further. This is usually followed by active exercises, so you can maintain the mobility the therapist has helped you achieve.

MUSCLE ENERGY TECHNIQUE. This is a distillation of physical therapy technique with elements of osteopathy and manual medicine. Your own muscle contractions are used to help realign and stabilize your torso, your back, and the rest of you.

STRAIN-COUNTERSTRAIN. Sometimes the body reports painful messages when they are no longer appropriate. Using the strain-counterstrain method, developed by an osteopath, your PT will put the painful muscle, joint, or area into a relaxed position. The muscle is shortened for 90 seconds to release it, then gently elongated throughout the muscle's range. The 90-second pause is meant to stop pain receptors from firing and allow the muscle to stretch and lengthen.

MYOFASCIAL RELEASE. The patient and therapist interact in the stretching process, the therapist receiving feedback for deciding the strength, timing, and type of stretch to effectively lower tension in the fascia, or connective tissue in the body. The therapist's touch may feel remarkably light but has powerful effects.

GAIT TRAINING. Analysis of bad habits or problems with walking—one-legged support, toe off, heel strike, et cetera—that could give you a backache.

CRANIOSACRAL THERAPY. A gentle, noninvasive, massage-like technique involving the bone plates that make up the skull. The theory behind the treatment is based on the principle that our bodies contain the means to heal themselves. The therapist "listens" to the body through palpation, then allows or introduces movement that will release restrictions caused by physical or emotional trauma.

MCKENZIE METHOD. Robin McKenzie, a physical therapist from New Zealand, developed a technique that has been proven by numerous studies to relieve back pain. Many physical therapists use the McKenzie exercises as a basis for much of the other work they do. For patients suffering from herniated disk, the exercises include movements such as side gliding and back extension. The McKenzie method is also somewhat analytic. Its goal is to identify the movements that produce pain, then shift that pain to the midline of the body through exercise, then reduce the pain, and finally eradicate it. An experienced physical therapist can teach some McKenzie techniques that you can do at home, and books on this method are available. These books emphasize self-treatment for back pain and provide prevention procedures.

DEVICES

TRACTION. This is designed to pull the vertebrae a safe distance apart from one another so that nerves are no longer compressed as they exit the spine. Theoretically, stretching the vertebrae apart by securing the feet and pulling at the top of the body should have a couple of good effects. First and most obviously, it should widen spaces in the neuroforamina so that possibly compressed nerves can travel in the space without as much trouble. Second, the muscle stretch provided by the traction sometimes relieves spasm. Third, when you pull two vertebrae apart, there is a greater volume of space, so the disk between them should bulge less and have an opportunity—provided by the partial vacuum—to be sucked back to where it's supposed to be, inside its healthy boundaries aligned with and between the vertebrae.

When traction involves the lower back, it is often not done to its fullest benefit, which can be achieved with force that is at least half the patient's body weight. Traction can be done for five minutes to half an hour, or in cycles, where pressure increases gradually, then decreases. After relaxation, another cycle of traction begins.

Though this traction method, which uses a harness at the top of the body and ankle straps, is done rather frequently, I believe that other methods of stretching the back are more effective. I think a simple forward bend is much more effective than a traction machine for stretching the muscles, separating the disks, and relaxing the lower back.

VAX-D. This machine allows a technician to control and monitor the amount of back stretch with a programmable logic controller located in a console. Continuous recording charts the activity of each cycle and may be printed for review by the treating physician. Some doctors have this machine available for their patients, and it may work reasonably well. However, a 2001 study in *Neurological Research* concluded that more double-blind, randomized studies were needed to prove its efficacy.

It is beyond the scope of this book to detail all the devices available to patients suffering from low back pain and sciatica. But here are a few of the most common, some of which I discussed in the section on what you can do at home.

LUMBOSACRAL CORSET OR BINDER. This external source of stabilization for weak musculature is a thick belt used for spondylolisthesis. It pulls in the abdomen, raising backward pressure in it. This pushes the vertebrae back, or at least keeps them from slipping.

INFLATABLE TRACTION. This wearable object goes from hips to ribs and works best for strong, big people. You put it on and pump up the air cells, creating more separation between your hips and your ribs. At the same time, this type of traction helps elongate the spine. At times I've seen it help when nothing else does.

ORTHOTICS. Tailor-made shoe inserts can change the way you carry your body, and alter the angle at which you stand. They can give you appropriate arch support so you have the correct foundation for the proper distribution of body weight, and they can also correct a leg length discrepancy. There are many types of orthotics with different purposes, such as improving knee motion, changing posture, and stabilizing a weakened ankle.

SIJ (SACROILIAC JOINT) BELT OR BRACE. This triangular padded belt fits over the sacrum and can be tightened below the iliac crest; it holds the sacrum together and may be helpful in treating sacroiliac joint derangement.

Many of the devices I've discussed can be obtained from surgical supply stores or from drugstores that specialize in this type of equipment. Usually your doctor or physical therapist will write a prescription for you; occasionally the specialists in the store will make sure you have the right thing. In the case of orthotics, a trained technician measures your feet and discusses your situation with your doctor or physical therapist, then makes exactly what you need.

Chapter VIII

MEDICATIONS

NONSTEROIDAL ANTI-INFLAMMATORIES

These drugs, in over-the-counter and prescription strength, are often given by physicians to relieve pain and reduce swelling—whether or not there is an official diagnosis—especially if the doctor suspects that the problem will resolve itself in a reasonable amount of time. Over-the-counter and prescription-strength Ibuprofen, Naproxen, and others decrease inflammation, swelling, and pain, as aspirin does. The first reason there are so many of these drugs is that there is lots of pain in the world. Second, sometimes one of these drugs but not another works on a particular individual, so if you've tried one and it hasn't helped, it's worth experimenting with others. Third, there is no way to determine which drug will be effective in a given situation, though some are definitely stronger than others, and some are less likely to cause gastric irritation.

In general, nonsteroidals are safe, but, like aspirin, they can cause stomach upset. It was this side effect of aspirin that made consumers look for alternatives and helped make Cox2 inhibitors, such as Vioxx, so popular. Painkillers such as Vioxx, Celebrex, Mobic, and Bextra were formulated to relieve acute pain just as well as other nonsteroidal anti-inflammatories but with a lower risk of gastrointestinal side effects and hemorrhage. These drugs were introduced in 1999, backed by more than $200 million in advertising dollars. Not surprisingly, the popularity of the Cox2 inhibitors soared. By early 2003, Vioxx and Celebrex together had sales of $4.4 billion. Vioxx, which many patients found especially helpful for pain relief, was the sixteenth most frequently prescribed drug at that time. But while people were taking these medications, researchers were conducting experiments to make sure that they were harmless. The bubble burst in 2004, when studies proved that some Cox2 inhibitors, although safer for the stomach than other nonsteroidals, were also more dangerous for the heart. Incidence of strokes and heart attacks went up for patients taking Vioxx for long periods of time. Merck, which manufactured the drug, voluntarily withdrew it from the market. Then, after further Food and Drug Administration (FDA) examination showing similar problems with other drugs, Merck said it would consider reintroducing the drug for specific patients for whom the benefits outweighed the risks. That's where it stands at this writing.

If you have a choice between prescription-strength nonsteroidals and over-the-counter products, I would suggest taking the former. Prescription-strength dosages are cheaper and safer. You need fewer pills, and those dissolve more slowly (because there is less surface area) and are less likely to cause stomach upset.

Should you have gastric problems, there are several nonsteroidals that can be administered in suppository form, or by injection.

Prescription-strength nonsteroidals don't contain narcotics. They are simply higher doses of a specific medicine, such as Voltaren. They do increase your tendency to bleed. But many narcotic preparations used postoperatively do contain non-narcotic painkillers in amounts that will not increase bleeding. Some of these are Percocet, Tylox, and Darvocet. In painful cases, these narcotic-Tylenol combinations are also good for pre-op or pre-epidural use, when the aim is to keep bleeding to a minimum. Another non-narcotic painkiller is Tramadol (Ultram), nearly as nontoxic as Tylenol. The dosage of Tramadol is slowly raised; its possible mode of operation is occupying pain-receptor sites in the brain. Its rare side effects are a little dizziness and light-headedness, which usually disappear with time.

Gabapentin (Neurontin) and Pregabalin (Lyrica) are anti-seizure medicines that we find effective for parasthesias, but not especially good for pain itself. Other medicines that are not specifically designed for back pain but are sometimes used for it are tricyclic antidepressants, which are often effective analgesics.

MUSCLE RELAXANTS

If your doctor believes that the source of your pain is muscle spasm or tightness, or that spasm or tightness is contributing to your pain, you will likely receive a prescription for a muscle relaxant such as cyclobenzaprine (brand name Flexeril) or carisoprodol (brand name Soma), which will help you feel more comfortable. Some physicians, because they believe that there is a muscular component to virtually all back pain, prescribe these drugs to almost anyone with severe back pain, as part of standard treatment. The muscle relaxant will help reduce the tightness or pull in the lumbar spine, where muscles may well have gone into spasm. In many cases, tight muscles actually pull the vertebrae together and further narrow the already limited space where an injury has taken place—where the nerve exits the spine. Studies have found that muscle relaxants can help a person who has acute low back pain.[44]

Investigators studying 1,633 patients who went to a variety of practitioners found that muscle relaxant use was not only common among those with acute low back pain, but their use was associated with more rapid recovery of function.[45]

Muscle relaxants are often used in combination with anti-inflammatory nonsteroidals, and I have found them somewhat effective in pain reduction. However, there are drawbacks. First, muscle relaxants are no substitute for finding out what's wrong. They treat the whole body rather than a specific, local problem. Hardly any muscle relaxant works directly on the muscles. Instead, these medications affect the central nervous system. This means they can be sedating, and in some cases moderately addictive. Patients complain that they would like to get out of bed but find it difficult when they're taking this type of medicine. I advise using these drugs cautiously, and not driving a car or operating heavy machinery. One way to minimize the unwanted drowsiness that muscle relaxants may cause is to use them at bedtime and take advantage of their sedating properties. Cyclobenzaprine is now available in half the dose formerly used, which seems to me to be just as effective as a muscle relaxant and much less sedating than the former strength. I advise patients to take one before dinner and another at bedtime. In the morning, if you are seeing halos around lights or feeling spacey, you can cut down on the dosage. If not, take three a day for a week. Most doctors limit the use of muscle relaxants to a week or so. One medicine does work on the muscles themselves—Dantrolene; unfortunately, its liver toxicity severely limits its clinical use.

OPIOIDS

This category of painkiller can be naturally derived from some form of opium or be synthetically produced. Whereas other nonaddictive painkillers are currently under development, opioids are the front line against severe pain. I usually prescribe Percocet for the first few days, then Oxycontin for more prolonged pain. These drugs work on the central nervous system, as muscle relaxants do. They are addictive, but mild and graduated dosing and withdrawal help reduce or prevent the cravings and withdrawal symptoms. Many patients fear becoming addicted, but unless they have a history of addiction, this is a worry that is not likely to come true.

When chronic, severe pain goes untreated or is inadequately treated, problems can also arise, and those problems can become permanent. Continuing, urgent pain signals from nerves can result in hypersensitivity in the injured area. The original location of the pain can widen. If you have chronic, unrelieved pain, it's a good idea to discuss the effects of specific drugs with your doctor, to make sure that you have long-lasting medicines as well as quick-acting ones to take care of breakthrough pain.[46]

PAIN MEDICATIONS ON THE HORIZON

Several promising new painkillers are now being studied or are just beginning to be used. One, called Prialt, is the first drug in a new class of non-opioid painkillers called N-type calcium channel blockers (NCCBs). This medication is targeted at treating chronic, severe pain. To avoid side effects, it is administered through a surgically implanted catheter directly into the fluid surrounding the spinal cord. According to the developers, Prialt is nonaddictive and 1,000 times more potent than morphine.

Other drugs that are on the drawing board as of this writing include bicifadine, which is similar to some antidepressants and is intended for low back pain. Another medication contains an opioid with an "antidote" aimed at preventing patients from becoming tolerant to it and also enabling the opioid in it to work better. Also being studied for their pain-relieving properties are marijuana derivatives, the active ingredient in chile peppers, and toxins from the puffer fish.[47]

As of this writing, the National Institutes of Health, in cooperation with Beth Israel Hospital in New York, is conducting a study to investigate the usefulness of Pamidronate for chronic low back pain. This drug has been used to treat bone pain by reducing the production of inflammatory agents that attack bones. It belongs to a class of drugs called bisphosphonates, which have been used to treat weak or brittle bones resulting from osteoporosis and other problems. Researchers have found the preliminary results with Pamidronate extremely promising. In a 2003 study done on subjects suffering from degenerative disk disease and sciatica, as well as other problems, 91 percent of those who tried this medication found pain relief.[48] Later research is even more encouraging.[49]

STEROIDS

We all have steroids coursing through our veins all the time, and we need them to live. President John Kennedy, who had Addison's disease and whose body didn't produce enough steroids, needed injections every day to make up for the deficiency. Normal people manufacture steroids, but when a doctor prescribes them for a specific reason, the amount is greater than your body makes.

Before taking steroids, you should know the cause of your pain. Steroids are generally prescribed for a herniated disk, other spinal nerve compression problems, and spinal stenosis. They are prescribed with the aim of reducing internal inflammation and swelling, and as an alternative to more invasive procedures, including surgery. The pain reduction that steroids provide opens a window for rehabilitation treatment, including physical therapy; or steroids can simply be used alone to reduce chronic pain. How do steroids work to help the pain—either chronic or acute—of a herniated disk? Basically, they decrease inflammation and swelling, which reduces painful pressure on nerve fibers.

This inflammation is caused by the movement of material from the borders or inside of the disk into the hollow tube inside the spinal canal where nerves are located. The body identifies this material as foreign and mounts a quick and intense immunological reaction. That means swelling, fluids collecting, irritants going there, white cells migrating to that spot, and everything reacting. All this happens in a space where there is no extra room, a space surrounded by bones and immovable cartilage. The swollen tissues press on nerves, causing pain and sciatica.

Steroids reduce that irritation. They can be given orally, or by injection. Both are effective, but each has its best use in different situations.

In my experience, oral steroids are actually a more radical treatment than injected steroids, because the medicine is disseminated throughout the entire body—including the liver, the kidneys, and the immune system—even though the medicine may actually be needed only between the fourth and fifth lumbar vertebrae. When patients take oral steroids, however, the medicine does get to the places where it's needed, as well as where it's not needed, and it generally does help.

When steroids are injected, it is usually close to or inside the central nervous system itself (the spine). This is both the strength and the weakness of the treatment. On the positive side, the medicine goes to the exact spot where the trouble is and doesn't have the side effects that are inevitable when it is distributed throughout the body. On the negative side is the necessity for getting the medicine close to the inflammation—often a tricky procedure that demands extremely accurate diagnostic information (supplied by the MRI and EMG) and considerable clinical skill.

The standard way of injecting the medicine is to try to place the steroid inside the spine so that it can spread out until it reaches the nerve roots. Another method is to inject the steroid outside but very close to the spine and at a specific level so it can work on the roots in that particular location. For some patients, steroids help for two or three months, then another injection is needed. This can be done, up to a point, but an individual's exposure to steroids should be controlled so the medicine doesn't create unwanted side effects. Some patients do have several steroid shots a year and find this treatment satisfactory for pain reduction. Some have one to three injections in a series and need nothing else for years, or ever. For still others, this treatment doesn't work at all.

There are so many contradictory articles debating the efficacy of oral and injected steroids that it's difficult to make an informed decision about whether to use them or some other treatment. I have found that injected steroids often have a stronger effect than oral steroids in reducing compression of nerves in the spinal column (stenosis) and nerves as they leave the spinal column (radiculopathy), but I think they must be injected at the proper spinal level.

If your physician suggests you try an epidural, it means that a trained pain expert or anesthesiologist will give you an injection of steroids near the site of the herniated disk or where the stenosis is most severely affecting nerve fiber function. Small shots of novocaine are used to numb the skin before the steroid is given. It actually hurts less than a vaccination against the flu, and most patients withstand the treatment well. When done with expertise by a physician, these injections bring good results as much as 70 percent of the time.

An excellent paper published in 2004 compared the results of epidural steroid injections with discectomy (removal of the herniated disk), and found that although epidural injections of steroids weren't as effective in reducing symptoms and disability resulting from a herniated disk, this type of injection could be helpful. Nearly half of the patients who didn't get relief from pain and sciatica after six weeks of noninvasive therapy did improve after having an injection—and they stayed better for three years. Still, patients who had undergone surgery had even better results, with up to 98 percent stating that the discectomy had been successful.[50]

Although steroids aren't for patients with diabetes (unless they watch their blood sugar carefully) or infectious conditions, or are immunocompromised or anticoagulated (taking Coumadin or Plavix), they are safe for a vast majority of patients when used correctly.

When all is said and done, studies of how well oral and injected steroids work are inconclusive. However, I tend to agree with an editorial in the *British Medical Journal*[51] suggesting that epidural injections may help reduce pain in the long term and the short term, and are effective in the management of sciatica that accompanies low back pain.

Over the past twenty-five years, I have prescribed oral steroids close to a thousand times and have noted that at least 50 percent of the patients get significant relief, with minimal side effects. One side effect I have noted, however, is occasional insomnia for the first two nights. I try to help patients avoid this by recommending that they take all the pills together in the morning rather than taking them at intervals throughout the day, which doesn't seem to reduce their effectiveness but does seem to alleviate sleeplessness.

Once in a while, oral steroids can make a person feel depressed for a day or two, or (more often) feel euphoric, yet nine out of ten of my patients experience no side effects at all. Some people worry that steroids can cause osteoporosis, which is a long-term concern, but one short course of oral medication or even a few courses of injected steroids will have only a minute effect on increasing osteoporosis. There are also rare cases where joints degenerate in a process called aseptic necrosis, alleged to occur after steroid use, but I have never seen this.

ANTIDEPRESSANTS

It's well known among physicians who treat back pain that low doses of antidepressants can be helpful—doses so small that they could not help with depression. Nobody seems to know why these medicines are so good for some patients, but this unusual outcome has been and continues to be studied. Researchers from the University of Washington in Seattle examined articles that appeared in medical journals assessing tricyclic and tetracyclic antidepressants for back pain. They concluded that these drugs appeared to "produce moderate symptom reductions for patients with chronic low back pain. SSRIs were less effective."[52]

Once, in the hall of a hospital associated with Harvard University, I overheard an exchange between two young psychiatrists, who marveled that when antidepressants were first formulated, there was disagreement about whether to call them analgesics or antidepressants, because their effects on pain modulation were as striking as their effects on mood. These drugs work on the central nervous system, affecting how a person perceives painful stimuli. Of course, antidepressants in small quantity or in any quantity don't get to the cause of the pain. In that way they're like Tylenol or narcotics. That's why I prescribe them so rarely.

My attempts to cure patients are always directed first toward finding out the cause of the pain, then working to remove that cause. When I prescribe antidepressants, I'm playing for time, aiming to relieve the person's discomfort while we get to the cause of the problem.

Chapter IX

INJECTIONS

EFFICIENCY IS THE NAME of the game when injections are used to deliver medication. In the case of a disease such as bacterial pneumonia, an injection of penicillin or other antibiotic disperses throughout the system from the muscle to which it is sent. When an injection is given to reduce pain and inflammation, the medication is often meant to go to the painful place and do its work right there.

Physicians injecting any substance into a painful muscle to relieve spasm are concerned with finding exactly the right location; accuracy is an issue. Two methods have been developed to reduce the possibility of injection inaccuracy. One of these involves using an EMG needle to help locate the right spot. The physician puts the needle into the area of difficulty, then asks the patient to move in such a way that the problem muscle is activated. If the read-out screen on the EMG machine doesn't show activation on the first try, the doctor tries a slightly different location until the EMG reflects activity when that muscle contracts. At that point the doctor has to employ knowledge of anatomy and kinesiology (physiology and the mechanics of movement) to make sure that the correct muscle and not some other one is responding.

This process sounds long and painful, but it really isn't. The physician usually comes close to the right spot in the first place; if not, the adjustments are small. I used this technique in a clinical study of a form of botulinim toxin for piriformis syndrome. My success rate in finding the correct injection site rose from 70 percent at the beginning of the study to 90 percent at the end, showing that the use of the EMG needle really did help improve injection site accuracy. After a short time I noticed another effect: I was hitting the right spot more often on the first try, which showed me that the technique is also self-teaching.

A second technique to improve the physician's ability to place an injection correctly is using a fluoroscopy machine and putting a radiopaque dye into the substance to be injected so that the placement of the medicine is clearly visible. This method is safe, gives a good image, and doesn't require much knowledge of anatomy or movement. The trouble with this technique is that the injection has to be completed before the physician knows where the dye went. Obviously it would be better to have exact knowledge of the site of the problem before giving an injection. Also, the dye itself, though it is usually harmless, can cause unpleasant sensations.

INJECTIONS FOR PIRIFORMIS SYNDROME

Enhanced MRIs were used by Aaron Filler and his associates at UCLA to find the precise location where an injection would do the most good. Using a titanium needle, which is not magnetic and doesn't interact with the MRI, up to thirty images were sometimes done before a single injection was given. After the injection was given, the MRI could be used again to see if the medicine was delivered by the needle to the right place. If not, Filler and his associates re-did the injection. This technique proved successful in getting to the place where the compression was occurring in piriformis syndrome.

Unfortunately, of the 162 patients who had MRI-assisted injections of Marcaine and steroid, only 23 percent experienced relief from disabling pain for more than eight months. Another 8 percent had a second injection, which gave them lasting relief.

Although MRI-assisted injection is a very new and promising way to help people who have piriformis syndrome, and although this research is well done, in my study of EMG-assisted injections of similar medications, 79 percent of our patients were 50 percent better for a period of ten months or more. This is more than three times the success rate of the California group.

The difference may be that we used physical therapy and rehabilitation techniques that not only stretch the muscle but help the patients become conscious of that muscle so they know how to relax it after the effects of the initial injection have worn off. It seems to me that the moments immediately following the injection provide an invaluable opportunity, and taking advantage of this window is imperative. Immediately after completing the injection, we give the patient physical therapy, including McKenzie technique, which frees up the roots of the sciatic nerve and gives it more room to move about. We make sure that the piriformis muscle stretches are done correctly by using assisted movement of the hip and manual stretch. Also, we use ultrasound and yoga exercises.[53]

After our first study, we made sure that each patient had two to three months of rehabilitation. Lately, using other agents such as Botox and Myoblock to relax the piriformis muscle, we found that 92 percent of the patients were at least 50 percent better after two to three weeks. For many of these individuals, whether they have rehabilitation for three weeks or three months, the exercises should be done at home, sometimes for years after the initial treatment. The physical therapy is essential for learning how to control the muscle. Yoga is excellent for gaining mastery over the muscle and its contraction. I have discussed the use of yoga for piriformis syndrome and sciatica from other causes in my book *Cure Back Pain with Yoga*.

OTHER TYPES OF INJECTIONS

Trigger point injections are usually given for various sorts of back and neck pain arising from muscle spasm but aren't given for sciatica. However, exactly the same type of injection is given in the piriformis muscle to reduce the spasm there. When this is done, it reduces symptoms of sciatica that occur when the piriformis muscle compresses the sciatic nerve.

This type of injection uses a combination of Lidocaine, a local anesthetic (which dulls the pain of the injection), and a very low dose of steroid. Why steroids work for muscle spasm is poorly understood; it's a question never answered to my satisfaction. I believe it has something to do with changing connections between surface membranes of muscle cells. The steroids may work to make muscle fibers less irritable and promote their coming to a resting state. Nevertheless, it has become standard procedure to use a bit of steroid to help relax muscle spasm.[54]

Marcaine is another medication often used in addition to or instead of Lidocaine. It's longer acting and is believed to seek out sensory nerve fibers and therefore be more effective than Lidocaine (which seeks out motor nerve fibers) in reducing pain. However, this medication can be toxic to the nervous system and to the heart, and must be used with great care.

Other medicines, such as Sarapin, are also injected. This totally natural material is derived from the carnivorous pitcher plant. It's not an anesthetic, but it is purported to have anti-inflammatory effects when injected into muscle tissue. I have used it a number of times, for example with diabetics, and found it effective in some cases and useless in others. Unfortunately little research has been done on this plant extract to define the best conditions for its use and its contraindications.

An injection is used to deliver sclerotherapy, a technique for treating sacroiliac joint derangement, which can lead to sciatica. Sclerotherapy purposely produces temporary inflammation and bruising. In this case the sugar or other unlikely ingredients that are injected are meant to produce a scar, which will eventually prevent the painful motion of a joint.

This sacroiliac joint injection may be done under fluoroscopy. Although it is beneficial for the doctor doing the injection to have a clear look at what is happening, I feel that caution is necessary here. The fluoroscope tells the doctor where the bones are, but it doesn't necessarily show where the real problem lies. I think fluoroscopy must be used after a good clinical exam that identifies the exact location of the greatest tenderness. Without that type of exam, the procedure may be safe but useless.

EPIDURAL INJECTIONS

Epidurals are slightly more invasive than the other injections we've discussed. An epidural, often of steroids, is an alternative to surgical treatment for severe lower back pain accompanied by sciatica that has not responded to physical therapy and less invasive treatment. In the past I had mixed feelings about the effectiveness of this relatively safe procedure, but now I have seen it work consistently for herniated disk, spinal stenosis, and degenerative disk disease when done by an experienced physician. When an epidural does relieve the pain of nerve compression, it allows the patient to take a more active part in a physical therapy regimen and also resume more daily activities.

Epidurals may be done by a physician in one of several specialties, including anesthesiologists and physiatrists. If you and your physician decide that an epidural injection is the right treatment for you, you will lie on your side or on your stomach on an X-ray table, and your doctor will place the needle, often using fluoroscopy for guidance. However, I have seen "old guard" physicians who have done thousands, even tens of thousands, of epidural injections with no muss, fuss, or bother, and no fluoroscopy.

There are two ways to deliver the epidural steroid: translaminar and transforaminal. The translaminar method gets the medication close to where the nerves are housed. The transforaminal method places the medication a little outside the space where the difficulty is, with the objective of diffusing it throughout the area, to reduce inflammation.

An epidural has the advantage of concentrating all the medicine in or near the spot where it is most likely to be helpful. If the medicine is not injected into the right location, you're better off with the global approach of oral steroids. Sometimes, when there are three or four problem spots in the spinal canal, as there may be with spinal stenosis, osteoarthritis, or multiple herniated disks, then the question of whether to use oral or injected steroids becomes more complicated.

There are cases of adverse side effects when steroids are injected, among them infection, nerve damage, and headache. Also, steroid epidurals are often not a permanent answer to severe pain and sciatica. If necessary, an epidural can be repeated up to three times a year.

IDET

Intradiscal electrothermal therapy (IDET) is a procedure in which a needle is used to introduce a wire into an injured disk, after which the wire is heated. The extreme heat destroys some disk material and reduces the volume of the disk. This procedure is meant to decompress nerves compromised by the disk. Respected researchers J. S. and J. A. Saal found that this method of treating sciatica that results from disk disease and has not responded to more conservative approaches "demonstrated a statistically significant and clinically meaningful improvement" in a follow-up study done in 2002.[55]

RADIO FREQUENCY ABLATION

This is another invasive technique addressing sciatica at its source—the sensory fibers of the affected nerve root. Using a Teflon needle and a fluoroscope, which shows exactly what is happening below the skin, an anesthesiologist places the tip of the needle at the location where damage must be corrected. The medial branch is a sensory nerve that is part of the posterior primary division of the nerve root. It serves the spinal muscles, the blood vessels, the sweat glands, the skin close to the spine, and the joints between one vertebra and the one above it and below it that is the target of that needle. Once the needle is placed, a type of electrical current reminiscent of a microwave is emitted from the tip of the needle for 1 1/2 to 2 minutes. This interrupts nerve conduction (and pain) and can actually inactivate the nerve root for up to a year or more. Pain is often diminished, even though the treatment has little effect on the functioning of the nerves to the muscles. Although the destruction of the nerve is permanent, as time goes on other nerve fibers appear and can grow into that space, and pain can begin again. At that point another procedure like the original one is sometimes indicated.

There are other techniques used to treat severe and unremitting sciatic pain that has not been cured by multiple surgeries or other interventions, but the necessity for these interventions is rare. One approach to extreme pain is a stimulator, which can be placed in the spine (in a minor surgical procedure) to sidetrack painful nerve signals and transform them into more innocuous signals. Other devices can actually deliver morphine into the central nervous system with a similar type of implanted mechanism.

Chapter X

SURGERY

OVERVIEW

When medications and other conservative treatments have failed, you and your doctor may agree that you need a more invasive procedure. Surgery is an option for some patients with lumbar spine problems, especially those with nerve pain going down the leg, or leg weakness. It can relieve pain as much as 70 percent of the time.[56] So, if you have a herniated disk or spinal stenosis, an operation may improve your condition dramatically. Several large studies report excellent surgical results for piriformis syndrome as well.[57] However, an operation may not work as well for people who suffer from low back pain without nerve involvement. Surgery for back pain alone satisfies the patient much less predictably—only between 50 and 70 percent of the time.

If you are considering an operation to relieve your chronic, severe low back pain and sciatica, it's important to make sure that you are a good candidate. Patients who benefit most from surgery are those who are carefully selected for an exact procedure. That means you have symptoms and there is diagnostic evidence that you have the problem for which you are getting your particular surgery. Don't laugh. Inappropriate surgeries are done sometimes, obviously without the desired results.

Ask questions if you are considering an operation. Look for a surgeon who specializes in spinal or piriformis surgery, and talk to your doctor about his or her experience with the surgery recommended for you. Get a complete description of the operation; don't settle for less than a full explanation of exactly what will be done, the chances of its success, and the details of recovery. Find out what can go wrong and, if something does go wrong, how it can be rectified. Then go further. If something does go wrong and needs to be fixed, what is the ultimate outcome likely to be? Any surgery is invasive, and can have complications. Try to balance the possibility of complications against the probable benefits in your particular case.

It's worth asking to speak to a patient who has undergone the operation you will have, with the surgeon you're considering using, so you can learn firsthand about the results. Due to the laws governing patient confidentiality, the way to do this is to have the physician's office ask the patient in question to call you. Satisfied patients (the ones your doctor will call) often cooperate.

It may be important to consult with your internist or other primary care physician to make sure you're physically able to withstand surgery.

In addition to the usual X-rays, MRIs, and other diagnostic tests, some physicians use the rather controversial discogram to determine whether it is the disk itself that is actually painful. This is done by trying to reproduce the person's back pain with an injection. As I've said before, a bulging or herniated disk shown on an MRI may not be responsible for the pain, but it often is.

PROCEDURES

For the right patient, surgery can be miraculous. In one case, a man I treated was in extreme pain but was frightened of going under the knife. Finally making the decision caused him almost as much anguish as the pain. But when he came out of the anesthesia, he said he could tell immediately, in spite of the pain of the recent incision, that the deeper, worse discomfort had already been relieved. Lying in his hospital bed, coming out of the anesthesia, this man already knew that the surgery had been a success. And this is a common story.

There are four basic surgical procedures to relieve nerve compression at a specific spinal level:

LAMINECTOMY. Removal of a small section of the bone that covers the nerve root and/or some of the disk material from beneath that root.

DISCECTOMY. Removal of some of the disk material from beneath the nerve root. After this operation, the nerve root has more space in which to heal.

FUSION. Joining one or more spinal vertebrae together so they no longer move.

ARTHROPLASTY. Repair of the joints between facets of adjacent vertebrae.

The procedure you choose will fall into one of two main categories. Although there are many techniques used to perform operations on the back, and many options, there are two main ways that the surgery is performed.

1. **CONVENTIONAL, "OPEN" SURGERY.** This is done with a regular incision. The surgeon looks into the wound to make the repair with or without a microscope or other visual tool. The patient needs recovery time in the hospital and at home, and often the pain resulting from the operation requires narcotics. Some surgeons believe that this type of surgery is preferable to the increasingly popular minimally invasive techniques, because it allows them to see and feel what is happening inside the patient rather than viewing it on a screen. The instruments designed for open procedures give the surgeon better control. Open surgery has been used for patients who have already had surgery; and it is best for complicated cases.

2. **MINIMALLY INVASIVE SURGERY.** This is done through tiny incisions—often under local anesthetic and often on an out-patient basis, with the use of miniature cameras, microscopes, and sometimes advanced imaging techniques that guide the surgeon. There are also various methods of achieving nerve decompression that can be done through tubes or even needle-like devices. Experts agree on the following advantages to this type of surgery.

* Fewer complications, except with microdiscectomy
* Less chance for infection
* Less loss of blood
* Less need for strong pain relievers after surgery
* Shorter hospital stay
* Quicker return to work and daily activities

However, make no mistake. Minimally invasive surgery is still surgery—the repair work done on the back is the same—and this type of surgery still requires recovery time.

There is consensus among experts that patients must be properly selected to benefit from minimally invasive surgery. For a herniated disk, the problem must be confirmed by an MRI or other imaging study. After about six to ten weeks of not responding to noninvasive treatments, patients who have herniation at one level, but with no evidence of stenosis, can be considered for this type of surgery.

As you can imagine, procedures that seem so quick, simple, and relatively inexpensive have their proponents, their detractors, and those who say that more study is needed. Dr. Franco Cerabona, head of orthopedic spinal surgery at St. Vincent's Medical Center in New York, believes that the decision to have minimally invasive or open surgery should be made on more than the idea that "it's just a Band-Aid over a 1-inch incision." "It's still invasive," he says of microsurgery. And it doesn't have a long-term track record. "If your surgeon isn't one who has done hundreds of these minimally invasive procedures a year, there's a chance that person won't be able to do it as well as the open procedure," says Dr. Cerebona.

SOME USEFUL MINIMAL SURGERY DEFINITIONS

MICRODISCECTOMY : A surgical procedure that removes a portion of a disk to relieve pressure on a nerve. Unlike a standard discectomy, it's performed through a small incision while the surgeon looks through a microscope. This type of surgery alters normal anatomy the least, and strives to maintain the patient's original anatomical structure. Most microdiscectomies are open, conventional surgeries. But there are modifications that are less invasive and are done through tubes and small incisions.

ENDOSCOPIC: The use of a tube containing small cameras and tools to remove parts of the herniated disk. The cable mounted on the camera connects to a TV screen, which displays the camera's field of focus. Also called percutaneous (see below) arthroscopic discectomy . The surgeon can see the disk and the nerve. At this writing, endoscopic surgeries have not been proven more effective than other procedures.

PERCUTANEOUS: Performed through the skin, such as the injection of radiopaque material in a radiological examination, or the removal of tissue for biopsy accomplished by a needle. Synonyms are transcutaneous, transdermal, transdermic. This kind of operation is like planes guided by radar; your surgeon cannot see the disk but looks at a real-time X-ray to see where the needle is going, and uses instruments to make the repair. The results are known after the surgery is completed and the patient is recovering.

There aren't a great many scientific studies on minimally invasive surgery, and the journal articles I've read are contradictory. One, done by researchers in the Department of Neurosurgery at Stanford University Medical Center and published in 2004, promises that further improvements in optics and imaging, development of biological agents, and the introduction of new instrument systems designed for minimally invasive procedures will certainly lead to more work in this field.[58]

Perhaps this method is more popular and trusted in Europe than in the United States. In Germany, a four-year follow-up of 200 patients found that percutaneous laser disk decompression (PLDD) is an effective and secure method to treat contained herniated disks. The advantages include the minimally invasive approach on an out-patient basis and a low complication rate.[59]

Italian doctors, studying 149 cases of herniated disk treated with this type of procedure, found that all patients had substantial relief. [60]

Newspaper ads along the lines of "End Back Pain Forever in 15 Minutes" often refer to laser procedures that are used in disk surgery to remove extra material that is pressing on nerves. The surgeons I know who do other sorts of back surgery are generally wary about this technique. They believe it's overrated, and although it does work from time to time, its success rate is not well documented.

There are a number of newer percutaneous disk procedures using small surgical instruments to remove or burn away disk material that may be pressing on nerves. These instruments can suction, cut, and burn (with lasers), and are used with the idea that if part or all of the nucleus, or inside of the disk, is gone, the disk will reabsorb any material that has escaped. More research is needed to prove that these procedures work.

Experts agree that most surgeons in metropolitan areas would give their patients the option of having a microdiscectomy rather than an open procedure. And there's a technique on the horizon that Dr. Cerebona believes is the wave of the future. When using it, the surgeon will employ a flexible fiber-optic tube with the diameter of a drinking straw. This long, flexible tube (called an arthroscope) has a miniature camera, a light, and precision tools at the end. It can enter the spine in the pathway of the affected nerve and follow that nerve into the spinal canal. It allows the surgeon to see the nerve, see the disk beside the nerve, remove what's necessary, then check to see that the area is sufficiently clear.

OTHER HERNIATED DISK PROCEDURES

Many different procedures, both open and minimally invasive, are available for patients with herniated disks that have produced severe pain and need repair. Two different approaches to this type of remediation are removing materials that compress nerve roots, and taking out the center portion of the disk to allow space for what has escaped to be drawn back in.

Chemonucleolysis was the first minimally invasive technique. It used injections of chymopapain (an extract of papaya) into the vertebral disk to treat patients with sciatica. This method quickly fell out of favor because patients experienced complications, some serious.

PERCUTANEOUS LASER DISCECTOMY. This surgery is performed by delivering a laser through a needle-like instrument to destroy parts of the protruding or herniated disk. It is a combination of percutaneous and endoscopic techniques. According to some experts,[61] most surgeons prefer monitoring the effects of the laser with a camera so the laser can be controlled, minimizing complications.

ARTHROSCOPIC MICRODISCECTOMY. Video-assisted minimally invasive surgery has been pioneered by Dr. Parviz Kambin, who has advocated its use for herniations involving the foramina—the openings through which spinal nerves pass. This is considered an attractive option, because the surgeon is actually looking at the nerve and can see whether the job is done. However, there is a learning curve for the surgeon; although patients do well in the short term, long-term results are yet to be established.

ENDOSCOPICALLY ASSISTED MICRODISCECTOMY. A tube with a light on the end is inserted into the problem area, allowing the surgeon to see where repair work must be done, and help in doing it.

LAPAROSCOPIC DISCECTOMY. This is a minimally invasive surgery done with tiny tubes of various types. The disk is reached through an incision in the belly.

There are many methods of disk surgery that use an indirect approach. Laser disk excision, suction discectomy, and percutaneous automated discectomy use a tube or a probe guided by X-ray to make the necessary repairs. The advantage to these types of surgery is little recovery time. But results of the surgery aren't known until later. Other, newer surgical techniques include the use of other tiny instruments augmented by fiber optics to identify the nerve root and remove any impinging disk or bone.

ARTIFICIAL DISK

At this writing, artificial lumbar vertebral disk replacements are in use in Europe; surgeons are looking forward to approval for their use in the United States. Artificial disks are appropriate primarily for patients who in the past would have been candidates for fusion. Disk replacement may help preserve spinal movement and avoid problems with disks above and below a fusion. There hasn't been time to test artificial disks over the long term, but preliminary reports in Europe show reasonably good results after ten years. Of course surgeons who will do disk replacements when FDA approval comes through will need special training. Down the road, technology will provide techniques for improving the various types of artificial disks already in use. They will be made of grafted cartilage or produced through genetic recombinant therapy. This would be enormously helpful for patients with severe degenerative problems. At this writing, artificial disks seem to be more successful in the mobile cervical spine than in the weight-bearing lumbar region.

SURGERY FOR PIRIFORMIS SYNDROME

When injections and physical therapy don't work for piriformis syndrome, surgery may relieve the pain, but I consider surgery a last resort for this condition. Surgery for piriformis syndrome may involve a range of different procedures. Sometimes all or part of the sciatic nerve goes through the muscle (rather than below it). In these cases the entire piriformis muscle must be removed. For most people, the muscle need only be thinned down and the area cleared of adhesions. The entire procedure takes about half an hour. In the last decade and a half, I've sent eighty-five patients who didn't do well enough with my usual treatment of injection and physical therapy for surgery, generally just for a thinning of the muscle and removal of debris to give the nerve free passage. This procedure is called neurolysis.

Only one patient, an ex-dancer (who had to have the muscle excised), complained of disability afterward; she could lift her leg without a problem, but once it was elevated she could not turn it out. This young mother was teaching ballet, and fortunately she could use the other leg to demonstrate to her students.

Within two to three weeks, the neurolysis patient is ready to resume all normal activities. I have seen only two cases of intermittent tingling in the leg after a patient had surgery, one lasting (with prolonged sitting) for eighteen months. Both of these patients had the less common excision procedure.

In our study, approximately 80 percent of the patients who had surgery had near complete recovery.[62] The same was true for Dr. Filler's group, though 3.7 percent of surgical patients and approximately one-third of injection patients in that research study showed signs of relapse after about four years amd four months, respectively. I believe it is the physical therapy and stretching exercises that have made more of the patients we have treated remain pain free.

UNNECESSARY SURGERY

Unfortunately I have seen many patients over the years who have been sent for surgery for a herniated disk when they actually had piriformis syndrome. One twenty-seven-year-old man in otherwise good health had a typical nightmarish experience. He had all the classic symptoms of piriformis syndrome—severe buttock pain on both sides—and sciatica, including tingling and numbness when sitting but not when lying down. But he didn't know what was causing his pain, and he had a great deal of difficulty getting a diagnosis. He sought the opinion of an orthopedic surgeon, who ordered two sets of MRIs and several X-rays. Though the MRI showed a slight bulging of the L5-S1 disk, there was no herniation. The patient had physical therapy and swam to strengthen his back muscles, without relief. He also had two epidural steroid injections, which didn't alleviate his pain either.

At that point, though the surgeon said he found it "hard to believe" that the slight bulging he had seen on the MRI could be causing the problem of buttock pain and sciatica, he advised the patient to have surgery. Thinking that the problem was in the young man's back, the physician recommended a spinal fusion. The difficult surgery necessitated a long and painful recovery. Six months later, having finally reduced the amount of narcotics he had been taking all along, the patient could feel enough to realize that he still had the same pain. When his original doctor suggested another surgery, the young man sought other opinions.

Finally, after ruling out problems with the spinal fusion and trying another round of injections, this fellow found out what he should have been told all along. Neither an operation on his back nor steroid injections in his back could ever cure him. There was nothing wrong with his back. At last he was given the correct diagnosis of piriformis syndrome. But his doctor was so unfamiliar with this condition that surgery was offered yet again. The man wisely chose a simple buttock injection and the proper physical therapy, and was 80 percent better within six weeks, albeit with a less flexible spine.

To me this is a cautionary tale. Beware. Do not settle for one opinion. Get two opinions, and if they differ, seek a tie-breaker. Find experienced doctors.

STENOSIS SURGERY

Minimally invasive procedures for stenosis are still being developed; as of this writing, there is no way to enter the spinal canal with tiny instruments and resect, or surgically remove, extra bone that is narrowing the canal and compressing nerves. However, the surgery that is available is often helpful. Because stenosis is progressive and more likely to be irreversible when it has gotten to the point that it is compressing the spinal cord, it is advisable to have surgery when you're younger rather than older. Though this condition may plateau and may move slowly, a person in his or her fifties can better withstand surgery than someone who is seventy.

Sometimes laser surgery is offered for stenosis, but it may not be advisable until it has been refined and studied, especially if you have cervical rather than lumbar stenosis.

FUSION FOR SPONDYLOLISTHESIS

There are different types of spondylolisthesis, which are described by different terms. You can have a problem where the vertebra is slipping forward, or where it is slipping backward, or where it is slipping forward in the upper part of the spine and backward in the lower spine. The most common type, however, is probably the degenerative spondylolisthesis that comes with growing older.

If you consider the spine as a stack of bones, one on top of the other, hollow at the center, it is easy to understand how the movement of one element forward would reduce the room inside the column. The joints of the bones that are stacked up in the spine sit right on top of exiting nerves, so if one bone moves forward even a tiny bit, the lower end of the joint will press on the nerve, causing pain and sciatica.

Key to deciding on fusion as an option for back pain is making sure that the instability or the movement of the disk is the actual cause of the pain. Paying close attention to the type of pain, what makes it worse or better, whether a back brace helps, and obvious abnormalities on X-rays and other diagnostic tests will help you make this decision. If a person needs to have surgery to remove bone that is compressing nerves (herniated disk or spinal stenosis), and spondylolisthesis is present, the fusion surgery that is done can be either open or minimally invasive. How much work to do inside the spine is the controversy—whether to add stabilizing hardware or to use a bone graft alone. Many experts believe that active young people who are walking around and engaged in normal activity and whose bones are strong may need screws or other hardware to supplement the fusion. Older individuals who may be relatively inactive and have weaker bones may not benefit from hardware.

There are several minimally invasive fusion procedures that are now in general use. Fusion can be done laparoscopically through the abdomen, and there are even some techniques that allow surgeons to do endoscopic fusions. Spine surgeons believe that the technology is improving, and many have inserted screws percutaneously.

Chapter XI

NONMEDICAL
TREATMENT
AND PREVENTION

THE RELAXATION RESPONSE

For individuals who suspect that stress is contributing to their back pain, various relaxation and meditation techniques can be extremely helpful. Herbert Benson, MD, a pioneer in mind/body medicine, has worked with the idea that physical symptoms are influenced by thoughts, feelings, and behaviors; also that physical symptoms such as pain can have a global effect on an individual—what he or she is thinking, feeling, and doing. Dr. Benson has defined the relaxation response—due to a simple form of meditation—and has done important research showing that a physical state of deep rest can slow the heart rate, lower blood pressure, and ease muscle tension. This demonstrably reduces stress and pain, which, research has shown, can have a long-lasting beneficial effect on a person's health. I have included one version of Dr. Benson's generic technique here, but there are many other ways to achieve the relaxation response.

Practice this once or twice a day in the morning and the evening. I believe that you will find it makes a difference to your overall health, whether or not your pain has an emotional component.

* Choose a word or a short phrase appropriate to your personal beliefs—for example, "peace," "shalom," "The Lord is my shepherd."
* Sit quietly in a comfortable position, eyes closed.
* Relax your muscles, starting at your feet and progressing to your calves, thighs, abdomen, shoulders, arms, hands, neck, and head.
* Breathe slowly and naturally; as you exhale, say your chosen word or phrase to yourself, focusing on it.
* If thoughts come into your mind, pay no attention to them. Just return to your chosen word or phrase.

Practice this for only 10 minutes. Then open your eyes, and sit quietly for another few moments. You can meditate once or twice a day for 10 minutes each time. Good times to do this exercise are before breakfast and before dinner.

JOHN SARNO

Dr. John Sarno's name has become almost synonymous with attention to the emotional aspect of back pain. Acceptance of the mind/body connection is growing in the medical community and the population at large, partly because of Dr. Sarno's influence. Unfortunately this idea has a long way to go before it becomes universally accepted and well understood.

In several seminal books (*Mind Over Back Pain*, *Healing Back Pain*, and the *Mindbody Prescription*), Sarno, a professor of clinical rehabilitation medicine at the New York University School of Medicine, has explained his theory that tension and unexpressed anger rather than structural problems fuel muscle spasms; the spasms affect blood and oxygen supply to muscles and result in pain. Sarno developed his theories because as a young physician treating back pain he found that he often had disappointing results. At the same time he noticed that many of his back pain patients had stress-related difficulties such as tension headaches, ulcers, and colitis. When he started paying attention to the emotional component of his patients' back pain, he had more treatment success.

Much medical literature supports Sarno's idea that in many cases low back pain and sciatica are related to psychosocial problems. Thousands of readers and patients swear by Sarno's theories and treatments, which include thought and behavior modification and, on occasion, psychotherapy.

YOGA

This ancient Indian physical and spiritual practice is now done by more than 20 million people in the United States. Hatha (physical) yoga consists of a series of physical poses, or *asanas*, meant to stretch the muscles, strengthen them, and improve overall balance. I myself have practiced yoga daily for more than a quarter century; for most of that time, I have used it therapeutically, with considerable success, to help my patients. I also have written about how yoga can help all kinds of back pain, including sciatica caused by disk problems in the back and by piriformis syndrome, in *Cure Back Pain with Yoga*.

Doing yoga doesn't cost much, involves very little equipment, and can be done by anyone of any age or skill level. Although it is connected with Hinduism, there are no priests. It promotes strength, flexibility, and balance; it can help you gain mastery over your own body by teaching you how to control your muscles; and it calms the mind. For me, yoga has become a way of life, and I highly recommend it to anyone who has back pain and sciatica, as well as to anyone who does not.

Some yoga therapists do nothing but help people with physical problems. I recommend looking into what they offer first. These therapists are trained to deal with all types of back pain and sciatica. The International Association of Yoga Therapists (IAYT) is one good resource (see Resources, page 186). Also, viniyoga is purely therapeutic and is done on a one-on-one basis (see American Viniyoga Institute, page 185).

Anusara yoga has helped many people (see below). There are other types of therapeutic yoga as well.

Ideally you should look for a yoga therapist or a teacher who has had a great deal of experience, is credentialed, and practices regularly himself or herself. Most important, make sure that your teacher knows the details of your back pain and your physical condition in general. Although yoga can be extremely beneficial for low back pain and sciatica, it is also possible to injure your back while doing it. Proceed with caution.

Yoga is an effective tool to control and cure piriformis syndrome. The stretches often bring immediate relief. If the easing of pain and other symptoms is not long lasting, the stretches can be done again and again. Make sure that you always do stretches on both sides. Yoga is also good for people who have sciatica and pain from herniated disk. In general, if you know that herniated disk is your problem, avoid twisting poses, which could aggravate the condition. Spinal stenosis also responds well to yoga, as does arthritis. Yoga can also be helpful for people who have had back surgery, speeding recovery and making the healing process more comfortable.[63]

If you have severe sciatica, discuss yoga with your doctor before starting it.

There are many styles of hatha (physical) yoga that are curative and preventative, but I do have preferences. Here are a few. Iyengar is the style of yoga I always practice. There are Iyengar certified teachers or an Iyengar institute in most major cities. The yoga they teach is anatomically sophisticated and therapeutically oriented, with a rigorous training and certification program that takes many years (www.bksiyengar.com; see also Resources, page 186). Anusara yoga is also particularly suited to people who have back pain and/or sciatica. It was developed by John Friend from work he did with the Iyengar style, with a focus on outer and inner body alignment and respect for each individual's limitations (see Resources, page 185). Kripalu is sometimes considered a good style of yoga for westerners and may help you begin to stretch safely (see Resources, page 186). Teachers of these and other styles of yoga must undergo training before being certified to teach.

Two extremely popular styles of yoga are Ashtanga, which is active and strenuous to the point of becoming aerobic, and Bikram yoga, which is a series of very active set poses done in a very hot studio. Before experimenting with these, I recommend that you try the styles of yoga I discussed above.

Meditation is intrinsic to yoga practice—another factor that can be helpful for anyone with a backache. Meditation produces the relaxation response that Herbert Benson and others have used so successfully. It calms the mind, helps individuals gain control over pain, and helps them cope with the stresses that may have contributed to starting the pain in the first place. I have found that meditation can inspire insight into the repressed anger and other emotions that John Sarno has identified as possible contributors to back pain. Meditation also helps create a sense of well-being.

ALEXANDER TECHNIQUE

This is a method of correcting problems with posture and movement, and relaxing tensions in the body with the goal of relieving pain and optimizing the efficiency with which individuals accomplish their daily activities. There is overlap and synergy between Alexander technique, physical therapy, Feldenkrais, Pilates, and yoga, all of which can be effective for backache and sciatica. According to an article by Alexander teachers Joan Arnold and Hope Gillman, the Alexander technique's premise is that the head must balance properly at the top of the lengthened spine without overwork or compression; problems arise, according to Alexander technique theory, when the relationship between the head and spine is poor.

I find that patients who are attuned to their own body do best with this system, because they are more easily able than others to become aware of unconscious tension and bad posture and movement habits, and to learn to take control of them until that control becomes automatic. Strength and balance increase gradually as the student behaves differently over time.

Alexander technique teachers work with students one-on-one, or in small groups, so they can provide a lot of individual attention, analyzing movement patterns, helping mobilize the body's central structural support system and reducing overuse and tension. The teacher uses a gentle, hands-on process to correct alignment and show the students how to sit, stand, walk, and perhaps accomplish other daily activities, such as sitting at the computer. The students need no special clothes for these sessions.

F. Matthais Alexander (1869–1955), an Australian actor, developed his technique for use as a training tool for other actors and for singers. Today his ideas remain popular with all types of performers. His technique also works well for athletes, pregnant women, and others with neck and back pain. Alexander technique is taught at the Julliard School in New York, the Royal Academy of Dramatic Art in London, and many colleges and universities.

PILATES

This method of strengthening the body's core is coming into the mainstream; physical therapists are incorporating it into their regimens, health clubs and spas offer it, athletes and dancers are fans. One of the advantages of Pilates is that it combines well with other strengthening, stretching, balancing techniques with which it shares some similarities, including yoga and Alexander technique. Pilates focuses on the core.

My patients who suffer from weakness, inflexibility, and muscle imbalance have found the Pilates method very effective. For some, such as those with scoliosis, more flexibility is not necessarily beneficial, and Pilates strengthening is too symmetrical to do them any good. But in general, when a person has a flaccid body, bad posture, and musculoskeletal problems, Pilates is a perfect solution.

The founder of the technique, German performer and boxer Joseph Pilates, took his ideas from his study of yoga, Zen, and ancient Greek and Roman physical regimens, making changes along the way. Around 1914, he began practicing his technique with exercises done on the floor. In surviving photographs of Pilates and his wife, one can see the beneficial effects of his specific type of regular exercise. The couple looks healthy and strong, even in old age. Pilates was interned with other German nationals in England at the beginning of World War I, and it was then that he invented the machines and props still used in the practice of his method.

According to the nonprofit Pilates Method Alliance (PMA), a primary focus of the work is deep, healthy breathing, which with regular practice results in increased lung capacity and better circulation. Another goal of the Pilates method is to strengthen muscles, particularly of the abdomen and back, and to make those muscles more flexible. Posture, balance, and core strength are essential to Pilates practice, and Pilates practitioners believe that conscious control of the body spills over into other areas of life, providing many other benefits. Pilates is not aerobic, though students often find the exercises strenuous. They praise this method as good for preventing all types of back pain. One of the elements I find beneficial in any bodywork method is also true of Pilates: there is teacher certification after a rigorous teacher training program.

FELDENKRAIS

Feldenkrais is allied with some other bodywork techniques—such as Alexander technique, massage, and chiropractic—in that there is hands-on work done by the teacher/practitioner on the student/patient. Feldenkrais maintains that what sets it apart from other methods is teaching people with physical limitations, such as chronic pain, to study how they move and to modify their movements to address the limitation. Neither an exercise system nor posture correction, Feldenkrais helps the student correct movement problems that he or she might not have been aware of. Automatic movements that may be causing the pain or contributing to it are identified, and substitute movements are taught.

The teacher evaluates movements, uses touch to examine the student, and looks for habits or patterns that could cause a problem. Bad movement habits can develop without an injury but can then cause one, according to Feldenkrais theory. Students learn privately and in groups, doing a series of gentle movements and sometimes actively assisted movement while being taught to regulate and coordinate their bodies. This is considered an educational rather than a medical approach; it helps students move without stressing affected joints to find comfortable ways to do what they want to do. When a student has a herniated disk or other problem that causes sciatica, the teacher will look for ways to help the student move less painfully, to be more comfortable, and to prevent future problems.

Chapter XII

NUTRITION AND LIFESTYLE

RESEARCH HAS SHOWN THAT above-average height and many hours spent driving are predictors for sciatica, and that sciatica may have risk factors that are separate from just a simple low back pain.[64] But proven or not, just about everything under the sun has been associated with back pain, including nutrition and lifestyle choices, such as smoking. Numerous studies verify that smoking is associated with back pain, because it causes "malnutrition" of spinal disks, resulting in damage to the cells in the annulus fibrosis (outer covering of the disk), and also damages the inner part of the disk, the nucleus pulposus. It's no surprise that the more nicotine your spinal disks are exposed to, the more likely it is to damage these delicate structures.[65]

NUTRITION

As for nutrition, excess weight makes backache worse, a fact I must sometimes bring to my patients' attention. Many of these individuals know that being overweight and having back pain go together like the proverbial horse and carriage. Still, that doesn't seem to motivate them enough to lose the extra pounds. In one classic case, a patient herniated one disk, kept making every meal a banquet, herniated another disk, and so on, until he had no choice but to change his eating habits or visit a surgeon.

Common sense says that carrying around too much poundage in front puts pressure on the sometimes fragile structures of the spine, not to mention the hips, knees, and feet. For many of my patients, it isn't actual obesity that's the problem. It's that ten to fifteen extra pounds that they lug through every minute of every waking hour. This weight eventually contributes to a breakdown of some mechanical structure in the back or a place that affects the back. I have always advised my patients to push their chair away from the table before they're completely full. Don't finish every morsel on your plate, but help control your weight by eating just a little less—5 to 10 percent—of everything. Exercise in general is useful for weight loss and for back pain.

It's also imperative to pay attention to eating a balanced diet that contains plenty of calcium for the health of your bones. Many people who have cut down on their intake of red meat (a source of calcium) to control their cholesterol level don't realize that they can add calcium to their diet by eating dark green leafy vegetables such as spinach and kale. Just one ounce of cooked dried beans—white beans or kidney beans, for example—provides 15 percent of your daily requirement of calcium, according to educational materials from the National Institutes of Health.[66]

Dietary supplements and herbal remedies—everything from fish oils to Chinese herbs to ginger—are purported to be cures for back pain, or at least for relief. There is a great deal of work to be done in this area, and some of it is under way at this writing.

Some research indicates that a combination of glucosamine, chondroitin, and manganese ascorbate may slow down degenerative joint disease, or osteoarthritis, particularly in the knee. These natural compounds were found to decrease pain and increase mobility and were well tolerated and safe in some studies. In 2000, an article in the *Journal of the American Medical Association*[67] found glucosamine and chondroitin reduced pain and medication use in osteoarthritis of the knee. Later work is still positive but substantially less dramatic.[68] It stands to reason that if a combination of these supplements helps the knee, it would likely retard the progress of osteoarthritis in the back as well.

I think these generally safe dietary supplements are worth a try, after a discussion with your physician, and if you buy a product that has standardized dosages. Use the supplement according to the package directions, and watch for side effects. Remember when taking any dietary supplement to find out whether it may interact with other supplements or drugs you are taking, and discuss that possibility with your physician and pharmacist.

LIFESTYLE

Your home and work environment—and the way you habitually use these places—can produce back pain, or can help relieve and prevent it. Watch for the patterns of your pain. What seems to produce it? Does your back ache after you've spent an hour reading in a specific chair or lying on the couch, watching TV? Do you have a good desk chair? Do you get up and move around often, whether you're at home or in the office? As my old friend Pyrrha says, "I try to keep moving. If I don't, I stiffen up."

Back pain can interrupt sleep, and sleeplessness can add to depression, which can worsen back pain. Here are some suggestions for dealing with sleeplessness:

* Check your mattress. If it's more than ten years old, you probably need a new one. Try it out in the store; it shouldn't be too soft or too hard. Many of my patients enthusiastically report that the high-tech mattresses that support the entire body have changed their lives for the better. These mattresses conform to the body. Where gravity pulls the most (from navel to knee), the mattress gives a little; it supports you where you need it the most (chest and sacrum). But try it before you buy it. I saw a patient recently who had bought an expensive mattress that turned out to hurt more than it helped.

* Use pillows. A patient of mine with stenosis had difficulty sleeping

until she experimented with pillows. After a great deal of trial and error, she found that sleeping on her back with a pillow tucked under her knees, and another one under her legs to keep them out straight a few inches above the mattress, was the solution. "It's not beautiful. I had to train myself," she says. "After months of pain and not sleeping, it was miraculous."

* Breathe. If you don't want to—or can't—take sleeping medications, do this simple breathing exercise, which has you breathing slowly instead of counting sheep. Stretch out in a comfortable position in bed, with the lights out and your eyes closed. Inhale slowly in three equal segments, stopping for a few seconds between each one. Your lungs will fill a little more with each part. Repeat this process 3 to 5 times. Now exhale slowly, reversing the way you inhaled, breaking up the exhalation into three equal segments. Your lungs will empty a little more with each portion. Repeat 3 to 5 times. You will feel relaxed, and you may yawn. This breathing exercise may work by raising the level of carbon dioxide in the brain, making you naturally sleepy.

* At your office, make sure your computer screen is at a comfortable eye level, directly in front of you and close enough so you don't have to lean forward to see it. If your back is aching, it is often extremely beneficial to take one foot off the floor, even a few inches. A footrest or a low stool can make a tremendous difference in your comfort level. Back support can also help. My wife never sits in her desk chair (or takes a long plane ride) without a lumbar pillow or support. This doesn't have to be anything fancy; it can even be a folded towel.

KINESIOLOGY

Modern kinesiology began in 1872, when Leland Stanford, governor of California, asked English photographer Eadweard Muybridge to determine whether a trotting horse ever had all four hooves off the ground at the same time. It took Muybridge seven years to prove, on film, that trotting horses did have free-floating moments. Eventually, he published an eleven-volume work entitled *Animal Locomotion*. This work is credited with starting kinesiology, which the American Academy of Kinesiology and Physical Education defines as "the study of movement and physical activity."

This field, used by OSHA (Occupational Safety and Health Administration) and ergonomists and physiatrists (doctors of physical medicine and rehabilitation) to understand adaptations to illness and injury, and by trainees in every sport, is also useful for investigating functional causes of back pain and sciatica.

Applied Kinesiology is a "pseudoscientific system of muscle testing and therapy," according to an article by Stephen Barrett, MD, on his consumer watchdog Web site. Although many chiropractors use this method, Dr. Barrett differentiates it from the true science of kinesiology, which is the study of movement and biomechanics.

BACK SCHOOLS

Patient education, often in an occupational setting, was introduced in 1969 and has been used since, with somewhat encouraging results.

The question is, what do back schools teach? This is not well defined or standardized, though back schools are sometimes part of a hospital, or may be incorporated within private clinics, and they are sometimes covered by disability insurance plans. A back school should teach a person how to deal with his or her chronic pain, how to recognize danger signs that make the pain worse, and how to maintain a healthy back through exercise. Students attending back schools are also advised about proper desk height, for example, and proper nutrition.

At the end of 2003, research studies of back schools were reassessed by looking at 3,584 patients with low back pain, without regard to whether they had sciatica. The evidence suggested that back schools do help, especially for individuals with chronic low back pain. These individuals returned to work more quickly than patients who didn't have the education. I am a believer in back schools, though I think that more research is needed to find out exactly how effective they are and how to make them more so.[69]

EXERCISE

There is wide agreement about staying active during bouts of back pain and sciatica. Lying in bed and doing little in the way of regular activities weakens muscles and slows recovery. Exercise not only helps relieve the pain, it aids in maintaining back health and is preventative. Almost anyone who has had severe back pain and has tried exercise is a convert. But what types of exercise are best? I believe in nonimpact, brisk movement that helps strengthen the body and keep the muscles supple. If exercise hurts your back, reduce its amount and vigor. Discuss what you can and cannot do with your physician.

SWIMMING. Water is an excellent medium in which to move; it is buoyant and discouraging of sudden, awkward movements. The backstroke, crawl, and breaststroke are good for increasing range of motion. The sidestroke poses little threat to an already injured back.

Scientific evidence strongly favors swimming for people with back pain. A Japanese study of thirty-five patients who did aquatic exercise and swam once, twice, or three times a week for seven weeks did well. More than 90 percent of the patients felt that they had improved after six months in the program, regardless of their initial ability in swimming. The results suggested that swimming may be one of the most useful modes of exercise for a patient with low back pain.[70]

BRISK WALKING. This activity, if done outdoors, can help change the context of your back pain by focusing your attention away from what's wrong. This aerobic, low-impact movement is also good for strength and flexibility. The American Association of Retired Persons recommends walking fifteen minutes a day, briskly enough so you feel your muscles working but not so quickly that you are winded. Walking not only helps relieve and prevent back pain, it may also help prevent hip fracture.[71]

Chapter XIII

ALTERNATIVE MEDICAL APPROACHES

Medicine used to have strict boundaries. If you had a backache, you went to an orthopedic surgeon or a specialist in physical medicine and rehabilitation. Any other practitioners were only considered by the lunatic fringe. Luckily, times have changed. At this point a person who has a back problem—or any other problem, for that matter—can choose from a wealth of treatment options that complement standard, old-fashioned conventional medicine.

The acknowledged connection between the mind and the body has created still more opportunities for healing. Americans have access to everything from acupuncture to guided imagery in the armamentarium for back pain, everything from nutritional supplements such as fish oils and Sam-e to tai chi.

Below is information I've collected about alternative therapies that may help anyone suffering from backache and sciatica.

OSTEOPATHY. Although osteopathy may be considered an alternative therapy, practitioners are educated in mainstream methods; doctors of osteopathy work alongside doctors with conventional MD degrees, and are well equipped to help anyone with back pain.

A doctor of osteopathy (DO) has been trained to look at the body as an integrated whole, with an emphasis on the musculoskeletal system—nerves, muscles, and bones. This fast-growing, family-practice-oriented, mainstream specialty offers all standard medical services, with a hands-on approach to medical problems. Osteopaths use ultrasound, heat, cold, range of motion, and postural adjustment in their treatment. During their four years of medical school, DOs learn osteopathic manipulative therapy (OMT), a technique involving hands-on diagnosis that I have seen work well for patients with back pain. Although OMT has sometimes been mistakenly compared to chiropractic adjustment, I find that it is more related to various physical therapy modalities, such as craniosacral manipulation.

ACUPUNCTURE. This 2,000-year-old Chinese medical treatment, one of the most widely used in the world, is increasingly popular in the United States, where an estimated 8.2 million adults have had the hair-thin needles inserted to relieve pain or another medical problem at least once. The question is, does it work for back pain? As with many other alternative therapies, more research is needed. However, a study funded by the National Center for Complementary and Alternative Medicine showed that acupuncture helps with pain relief and improves function in people with osteoarthritis of the knee. It can be used effectively along with conventional care, and it may be a valuable addition to standard care for individuals with back pain, osteoarthritis, and other problems. Another PET-scan study showed the parts of the brain (insula ipsilaterale) excited by acupuncture, but not by placebo.[72]

Although there are written requirements for becoming a certified acupuncturist in about forty states, they are not standardized. Nor does a license guarantee expertise. If your acupuncturist gives you a diagnosis, I recommend augmenting it with a second opinion from a physician. Acupuncture treatments are often reimbursed by health insurance.

CHIROPRACTIC. This form of treatment—one of the "manual therapies," which was founded in 1895 by David Palmer—has never been more popular, especially for back pain. Patients made an estimated 192 million visits to chiropractors in the United States in 1997, according to the National Center for Complementary and Alternative Medicine. Patients report very high levels of satisfaction with chiropractic care, which consists in large part of manipulating the spine to alleviate subluxation (partial dislocation, as in one of the bones in a joint). The manipulations are called "adjustments." They are performed mainly on the spine, where the chiropractor applies a specific, sudden force to a joint, with the goal of increasing range of motion and relieving pain. Chiropractors are quick to point out that they don't dispense drugs or do surgery, rather they treat patients conservatively. They are considered "doctors" under Medicare and in a majority of states, and many health insurance plans reimburse for chiropractic treatments.

There are conflicting reports about whether it's less effective and/or less expensive to visit a chiropractor rather than an MD, but some research has been done to make an objective determination. Expense is, of course, one of the factors that could help patients decide whether to see a chiropractor or another health care professional. As for how well chiropractic works, highly respected scientists compared the results of physical therapy, chiropractic, and an educational booklet, and reported that patients who saw a physical therapist or a chiropractor had similar results, which were just a little bit better than giving the individual with the backache an educational booklet on how to care for the back.[73] (Another study of 682 patients with low back pain found that after six months the results of chiropractic care and care by a conventional medical doctor were more or less the same, though there was a slight extra benefit for patients who saw a doctor and received physical therapy.)[74]

Chiropractors must graduate from a four-year program, then take a state licensing exam in order to practice. There are possibilities for postgraduate training, including specialization in residency programs lasting two or three years.

With any health care practitioner, the quality of care you receive may vary tremendously, depending on the talent and skills of the individual who is treating you. Many people swear by their chiropractors. I believe that the chiropractor's use of X-ray may not always be as helpful in the diagnosis and subsequent treatment of sciatica as the MRI and EMG and a thorough, informed physical exam.

HOMEOPATHY. This European system of medicine became popular in the United States in the nineteenth century, then died out, and is now experiencing a resurgence. When you are ill or have a backache or even emotional difficulties, a homeopathic doctor tries to stimulate your body to cure itself by administering specific medications that produce the same symptoms. Symptoms are seen as the body's way of expressing its need to help itself. If you have a cough, a homeopath won't try to suppress it with cough medicine but will give you something that would stimulate a cough in a healthy person; the idea is that matching the symptom to the substance that can mimic it will bring on a cure.

Homeopathic remedies are monitored by the FDA, and several are recommended for the pain of sciatica and other backache. Although there are many skilled homeopaths, and some patients have complete trust in their remedies, this specialty is largely unregulated, and an individual can rather quickly and easily obtain credentials to practice it. However, many MDs and ODs also study and administer homeopathic remedies.

BODYWORK. In the alternative medicine environment that has grown up in the past twenty-five years, many people best called bodyworkers are now using a wide variety of techniques, ranging from kinetic awareness—used by people of significant sophistication—to techniques they developed on their own. In a previous career, these bodyworkers may have been chiropractors or PTs or dancers or trainers; they found ways to cure their own ills or those of their colleagues, and then applied them. Some of these people have a good deal of general scientific and biological learning; others have practically none. Their background goes from formal education to things they've picked up almost anecdotally, certainly empirically from what they've actually done. In general they're the most diffuse group I can think of, and it's impossible to pass judgment on them. It would be like passing judgment on houses, from McMansions to shacks. But in general I wouldn't consult an unlicensed bodyworker without a doctor's advice.

REIKI. This is an ancient energy technique with a spiritual component directed at helping the whole patient, not just relieving a specific
medical condition. However, a colleague of mine, an MD who is a pain
management specialist, regularly calls a reiki master to help with difficult cases. Reiki is said to promote healing. It is a stress reducer with
cumulative effects and is used to help a wide range of complaints, from
anxiety to insomnia, from pain relief to reducing the side effects of prescription medications. Reiki is safe and low cost, and can be self-
administered after it is learned.

A reiki session consists of the fully dressed patient sitting or lying
comfortably and receiving light touch from the reiki master. He or she
usually touches the head, the front, and the back of the person receiving
the reiki. This touch can also be applied directly to the injury or problem
area.

High-quality research to determine the effectiveness of this technique
is being done under the auspices of the National Center for Complementary and Alternative Medicine. Reiki is often used in addition to
conventional medical techniques, such as chemotherapy, and can also
be combined with acupuncture, chiropractic, homeopathy, or other
alternative techniques.

FELDENKRAIS METHOD. This bodywork method, based on the
ideas of Moshe Feldenkrais (1904–1984), an engineer, physicist, inven-
tor, and judo expert, is designed for people who have chronic pain,
restricted movement, and psychological or neurological problems, as
well as for performing artists and athletes. The method is based on the
idea that individuals naturally learn to function on a physical level, but
not necessarily at an optimum level. One of the goals of Feldenkrais is to
help people improve basic functional skills, such as walking and sitting.
The work itself is meant to be relaxing, painless, and no-impact, with
emphasis on alignment and range of motion—issues that often need to
be addressed to help relieve back pain.

"Functional integration" is Feldenkrais treatment that is tailored to
the individual. The client lies or sits on a specially designed table, comfortably and fully dressed, while the practitioner guides him or her

through a series of movements that are designed to break bad habits and retrain the nervous system. Props are sometimes used.

Group instruction, "Awareness Through Movement," usually lasts from 30 to 60 minutes and emphasizes a specific function. Group members perform movements based on everyday activities or on the relationship between specific joints, muscles, and posture, trying to become more aware of old habits and increasing their sensitivity to new ones.

Feldenkrais is designed for people of all ability levels. I have seen this method help people with backache and sciatica and also other conditions. The International Feldenkrais Federation (IFF) is an umbrella organization for most Feldenkrais guilds and associations. Certified instructors must graduate from a Feldenkrais guild accredited program, a process that requires forty days of study per year and usually takes four years.

MASSAGE THERAPY. If you have severe backache and sciatica and know where your injury is, you can have massage, but it should be administered with extreme caution, and you should carefully protect yourself by making sure that there is no pressure or movement directly on the injury. Have as much massage as you want, and of any type, as long as there is no manipulation of the exact spot where your pain originates.

There are many other techniques that use pressure and movement to manipulate the body, provide relaxation and ease discomfort.[75] Here are a few.

AYURVEDIC MASSAGE. Gentle and soothing, it is by definition meant to be healing.

SHIATSU. This traditional Japanese massage therapy is done with fingertips and palms, sometimes rather forcibly, at acupuncture points. It may be used to relieve pain, tension, and arthritis.

SWEDISH MASSAGE. The most common type of massage done in health clubs and spas, this is often done over most of the body, and consists of several manipulations, including rubbing, kneading, and tapping. Usually this style of massage is pleasant and can be therapeutic.

REFLEXOLOGY. This technique is said to help relieve pain when points on the hands and feet that correspond to other areas of the body are linked with other body parts. Personally I find it difficult to accept that reflexology can be useful to patients with back pain and sciatica.

TUI NA. In this technique, pressure is applied with the fingers and thumb, and specific points on the body (acupoints) are manipulated.

TAI CHI. All across China every morning, groups of older people congregate in public parks to keep themselves fit by doing tai chi, the ancient Chinese practice of 108 movements based on the teachings meant to promote physical and spiritual health. Like many other good mind/body practices, tai chi (and its cousin qi gong) is beneficial for strength, balance, and flexibility. Although tai chi may not directly alleviate sciatica, it could have indirect beneficial effects.

According to the International Taoist Tai Chi Society, tai chi movements include relaxation, balance, lining up the body, correcting angles, "squaring" the hips, controlling the step and the transfer of weight, turning constantly in spirals, "opening" and "closing," centering the trunk, and stretching and relaxing the spine.[76]

Several scientific studies have attempted to quantify the benefits of tai chi. Researchers in Boston, reviewing the literature, found that tai chi "appears to have physiological and psychosocial benefits and also appears to be safe and effective in promoting balance control, flexibility, and cardiovascular fitness in older patients with chronic conditions" but concluded that more study is needed before the benefits, if any, of this ancient art are fully known.[77]

NOTES

Chapter I

1. X. Luo, R. Pietrobon, et al. "Estimates and patterns of direct health care expenditures among individuals with back pain in the United States," *Spine* 29, no. 1 (January 1, 2004): 79–86.
2. M. Heliovaara, M. Makela, M. Knekt, et al. "Determinants of sciatica and low back pain," *Spine* 16, no. 6 (June 1991): 608–14.
3. A. Leclerc, F. Tubach, et al. "Personal and occupational predictors of sciatica in the GAZEL cohort," *Occupational Medicine* (London) 53, no. 6 (September 2003): 384–91.
4. Aaron Filler, J. Haynes, S. E. Jordan, and J. Prager. "Sciatica of nondisc origin and piriformis syndrome: diagnosis by magnetic resonance neurography and interventional magnetic resonance imaging with outcome study of resulting treatment," *Journal of Neurosurgery: Spine* 2 (2005): 99–115.
5. Roger P. Hallin. "Sciatic pain and the piriformis muscle," *Postgraduate Medicine* 74, no. 2 (1983): 69–74.
6. Filler, et al. *Journal of Neurosurgery: Spine.*
7. D. M. Long, M. BenDebba, et al. "Persistent back pain and sciatica in the United States: patient characteristics," *Journal of Spinal Disorders* 9, no. 1 (February 1996): 40–58.
8. D. L. Patrick, R. A. Deyo, et al. "Assessing health-related quality of life in patients with sciatica," *Spine* 20 (September 1, 1995): 1899–1908.
9. Agency for Health Care Policy and Research. *Acute Low Back Problems in Adults,* Clinical Practice Guideline no. 14, Rockville, Md. (1994): Publication 95-0642.

10. S. J. Atlas, R. B. Keller, Y. Chang, et al. "Surgical and nonsurgical management of sciatica secondary to a lumbar disc herniation: five-year outcomes from the Maine Lumbar Spine Study," *Spine* 26, no. 10 (May 15, 2001): 1179–87.

11. A. L. Dunn, R. E. Andersen, and J. M. Jakicic. "Lifestyle physical activity interventions. History, short- and long-term effects, and recommendations," *American Journal of Preventative Medicine* 15, no. 4 (November 1998): 398–412.

12. K. B. Hagen, et al. "The Cochrane review of advice to stay active as a single treatment for low back pain and sciatica," *Spine* 27, no. 16 (August 15, 2002): 1736–41, review.

13. I. Karamplas, A. Boev III, and N. Kostas. "Sciatica: a historical perspective on early views of a distinct medical syndrome," *Neurosurgical Focus* 16 (January 2004).

14. R. C. Parisien, P. A. Ball, and William Jason Mixter. "Ushering in the 'dynasty of the disc,'" *Spine* 23 (1998): 2363–6.

Chapter II

15. Filler, et al. *Journal of Neurosurgery: Spine*.

16. N. Boos, S. Weissback, et al. "Classification of age-related changes in lumbar intervertebral discs," 2002 Volvo Award in basic science, *Spine* 27, no. 23 (December 1, 2002): 2631–44.

17. J. Audette. "Botulinim Toxin Type B injection for a patient with myofascial pain," *Pain Medicine* 3, no. 2 (June 2002): 174–5.

18. M. Jensen. "Magnetic resonance imaging of the lumbar spine in people without back pain," *New England Journal of Medicine* 331, no. 2 (July 14, 1994): 69–73.

19. G. K. Lutz, M. E. Butzalaff, et al. "The relation between expectations and outcomes in surgery for sciatica," *Journal of General Internal Medicine* 14 (December 1999): 740–4.

Chapter III

20. Filler, et al. *Journal of Neurosurgery: Spine*.
21. *Ibid.*

Chapter IV

22. K. D. Johnsson and M. Sass. "Cauda equina syndrome in lumbar spinal stenosis: case report and incidence in Jutland, Denmark," *Journal of Spinal Disorders and Techniques* 17, no. 4 (August 2004): 334–5.

23. Jensen. *New England Journal of Medicine*.

Chapter V

24. Filler, et al. *Journal of Neurosurgery: Spine.*

25. Jensen. *New England Journal of Medicine.*

26. Agency for Health Care Policy and Research. *Acute Low Back Problems in Adults.*

27. *Ibid.*

28. www.americanrunning.org./displayindustryarticle.cfm?articlenbr=2056.

29. www.ninds.nih.gov/health_and_medical_disorders/piriformis_syndrome.htm.

30. E. C. Papadropoulos and S. N. Khan. "Piriformis syndrome and low back pain: a new classification and review of the literature," *Orthopedic Clinics of North America* 35, no. 1 (January 2004): 65–71.

31. Filler, et al. *Journal of Neurosurgery: Spine,* 114.

32. L. M. Fishman and P. A. Zybert. "Electrophysiological evidence of piriformis syndrome," *Archives of Physical Medicine and Rehabilitation* 73 (April 1992): 359–64.

33. L. M. Fishman. "Electrophysiological evidence of piriformis syndrome," *Archives of Physical Medicine and Rehabilitation* 69 (1988): 800, abstract.

34. L. M. Fishman and M. Schaefer. "The piriformis syndrome is underdiagnosed," *Muscle and Nerve* (November 2003): 626–9.

35. C. A. McTomoney and L. J. Micheli. "Current evaluation and management of spondylolysis and spondylolisthesis," *Current Sports Medicine Report* 2, no. 1 (February 2003): 41–6.

36. E. Vlaanderen, N. E. Conza, C. J. Snijders, A. Bouakaz, and N. De Jong. "Low back pain, the stiffness of the sacroiliac joint: a new method using ultrasound," *Ultrasound in Medical Biology* 31, no. 1 (January 2005): 39–44.

37. T. Shih and J. J. Lynn. "Lumbar zygapophypseal joint injections in patients with chronic low back pain," *Journal of the Chinese Medical Association* 68, no. 2 (February 2005): 59–64.

38. D. A. Mayer, R. J. Gatchel, et al. "A randomized clinical trial of treatment for lumbar segmental rigidity," *Spine* 29, no. 20 (October 15, 2004): 2199–205, discussion 2206.

39. *Ibid.*

40. V. Mooney and J. Robertson. "Radio frequency ablation is effective in recalcitrant cases," *Clinical Orthopaedics* 115 (March–April 1976): 149–56.

Chapter VI

41. www.osha.gov/SLTC/ergonomics.

42. S. Schaffer and C. B. Yucha. "Relaxation and pain management: the relaxation response can play a role in managing chronic and acute pain," *American Journal of Nursing* 104, no. 8 (August 2004): 75, 76, 78, 79, 81, 82.

Chapter VII

43. S. F. Nadler, et al. "Overnight use of continuous low-level heatwrap therapy for relief of low back pain," *Archives of Physical Medicine and Rehabilitation* 84, no. 3 (March 2003): 335–42.

Chapter VIII

44. T. J. Schnitzer, et al. "A comprehensive review of clinical trials on the efficacy and safety of drugs for the treatment of low back pain," *Journal of Pain and Symptom Management* 28, no. 1 (July 2004): 72–95.

45. E. Bernstein, et al. "The use of muscle relaxant medications in acute low back pain," *Spine* 29, no. 12 (June 15, 2004): 1346–51.

46. Jane Brody. Personal Health. "Some side effects of opioids include upset stomach, dizziness, and constipation," *New York Times* (February 15, 2005): Section F.

47. Andrew Pollack. "The search for the killer painkiller," *New York Times* (February 15, 2005): Section F, page 1.

48. M. Pappagallo, B. Breuer, A. Schneider, and K. J. Sperber. "Treatment of chronic mechanical spinal pain with intravenous pamidronate: a review of medical records," *Journal of Pain and Symptom Management* 26, no. 1 (July 2003): 678–83.

49. J. Rittweger, H. M. Frost, et al. "Muscle atrophy and bone loss after 90 days' bed rest and the effects of flywheel resistive exercise and pamidronate: results from the LTBR study," *Bone* 36, no. 6 (June 2005): 1019–29.

50. G. Buttermann. "Treatment of lumbar disc herniation: epidural steroid injection compared with discectomy, a prospective, randomized study," *Journal of Bone and Joint Surgery* V86A, no. 4 (April 2004).

51. A. Samanta and J. Samanta. "Is epidural injection of steroids effective for low back pain?" *British Medical Journal* 328 (June 26, 2004): 1509–10.

52. T. O. Staiger, B. Gaster, et al. "Systematic review of antidepressants in the treatment of chronic low back pain," *Spine* 28, no. 22 (November 15, 2003): 2540–5.

Chapter IX

53. Loren Fishman, et al. "Piriformis syndrome: diagnosis, treatment, and outcome—a 10-year study," *Archives of Physical Medicine and Rehabilitation* 83, no. 3 (March 2002): 295–301, review.

54. C. Steiner, C. Staubs, M. Ganon, and L. Buhlinger. "Piriformis syndrome:

pathogenesis, diagnosis, and treatment," *Journal of the American Osteopathic Association* 87 (1987): 318–23.

55. B. Freedman, S. Cohen, T. R. Kuklo, et al. "Intradiscal electrothermal treatment for chronic discogenic low back pain: prospective outcome study with a minimum 2-year follow-up," *Spine* 27, no. 9 (May 1, 2002): 966–73, discussion 973–4.

Chapter X

56. S. J. Atlas, R. B. Keller, Y. A. Wu, R. A. Deyo, and D. E. Singer. "Long-term outcomes of surgical and nonsurgical management of sciatica secondary to a lumbar disc herniation: 10 year results from the Maine Lumbar Spine Study," *Spine* 30, no. 8 (April 15, 2005): 927–35.

57. Loren Fishman, et al. *Archives of Physical Medicine and Rehabilitation.*

58. I. Thongtrangan, H. Le, J. Park, and D. H. Kim. "Minimally invasive spinal surgery: a historical perspective," *Neurosurgical Focus* 16, no. 1 (January 15, 2004): E13.

59. D. H. Gronemeyer, H. Buschkamp, M. Braun, S. Schirp, et al. "Image-guided percutaneous laser disk decompression for herniated lumbar disks: a 4-year follow-up in 200 patients," *Journal of Clinical Laser Medicine and Surgery* 21, no. 3 (June 2003): 131–8.

60. A. Latorraca, N. Forni, and C. Gamba. "Analysis on 149 consecutive cases of intervertebral lumbar and cervical disc prolapse operated with microendoscopic (Metr'X) technique," *Reumatismo* 56, no. 1 (January–March 2004): 31. In Italian.

61. M. Savitz, J. Chiu, and A. Yeung. "Percutaneous Laser Discectomy, The Practice of Minimally Invasive Spinal Technique," *AAMISMS Education* LLC (2000): 100–103.

62. Loren Fishman, et al. *Archives of Physical Medicine and Rehabilitation.*

Chapter XI

63. K. J. Sherman, D. C. Cherkin, et al. "Comparing yoga, exercise, and a self-care book for chronic low back pain: a randomized, controlled trial." *Annals of Internal Medicine* (December 20, 2005): 849–56; and K. A. Williams, et al. "Effect of Iyengar yoga therapy for chronic low back pain." *Pain* (May 2005): 107–17.

Chapter XII

64. A. Leclerc, et al. *Occupational Medicine* (London).

65. M. Akmal, et al. "Effect of nicotine on spinal disc cells: a cellular mechanism for disc degeneration," *Spine* 29, no. 500 (March 1, 2004): 568–75.

66. www.ama-cmeonline.com/pain_mgmt/module08/05osteo/06_01.html.

67. T. E. McAlindon, et al. "Glucosamine and chondroitin for treatment of osteoarthritis: a systematic quality assessment and meta-analysis," *Journal of the American Medical Association* 283 (2000): 1469–75.

68. D. O. Clegg, D. J. Reda, C. L. Harris, et al. "Glucosamine, chondroitin sulfate, and the two in combination for painful knee osteoarthritis," *New England Journal of Medicine* 354 no. 8 (February 23, 2006): 858–60.

69. M. W. Heymans, M. W. van Tulder, et al. "Back schools for nonspecific low back pain: a systematic review within the framework of the Cochrane Collaboration Back Review Group," *Spine* 30, no. 19 (October 1, 2005): 2153–63.

70. M. Ariyoshi, et al. "Efficacy of aquatic exercises for patients with low back pain," *Krume Medical Journal* 46, no. 2 (1999): 91–6.

71. www.aarp.org/health-active/walking/Articles/a2004-06-17-walking-numerousbenefits.html, accessed August 15, 2005.

Chapter XIII

72. www.pdrhealth.com/content/natural_medicine/chapters/201400.shtml.

73. D. C. Cherkin, R. A. Deyo, M. Battie, et al. "A comparison of physical therapy, chiropractic manipulation," *Spine* 27, no. 13 (July 1, 2002): 1476–7.

74. E. L. Hurtwitz, et al. "A randomized trial of medical care with and without physical therapy and chiropractic care with and without physical modalities for patients with low back pain: 6-month follow-up outcomes from the UCLA low back pain study," *Spine* 27, no. 18 (October 15, 2002): 2193–204.

75. nccam.nih.gov/health/backgrounds/manipulative.

76. www.taoist.org/english.

77. C. Wang, J. Collet, and J. Lau. "The effect of tai chi on health outcomes in patients with chronic conditions: a systematic review," *Archives of Internal Medicine* 164 (2004): 493–501.

resources

American Academy of Orthopaedic
  Surgeons
6300 North River Road
Rosemont, Illinois 60018-4262
847-823-7186 or 800-346-AAOS
Fax: 847-823-8125
www.aaos.org

American Society for the Alexander
  Technique
P.O. Box 60008
Florence, Massachusetts 01062
800-473-0620 or 413-584-2359
Fax: 413-584-3097
www.alexandertech.org

American Viniyoga Institute
P.O. Box 88
Makawao, Hawaii 96768
808-572-1414
Fax: 808-573-2000
www.viniyoga.com

Anusara (yoga)
9400 Grogan's Mill Road, Suite 200
The Woodlands, Texas 77380
888-398-9642 or 281-367-9763
Fax: 281-367-2744
www.anusara.com

Georgia State University Department of Kinesiology and Health
Georgia State University
University Plaza
Atlanta, Georgia 30033-3083
404-651-2536
www.gsu.edu/kin

Herbert Benson
Mind/Body Medical Institute
824 Boylston Street
Chestnut Hill, Massachusetts 02467
617-991-0102 or 866-509-0732
Fax: 617-991-0112
www.mbmi.org

International Association of Yoga
  Therapists
115 S. McCormick Street, Suite 3
Prescott, Arizona 86303
928-541-0004
Fax: 928-541-9182
www.iayt.org

International Feldenkrais Federation
www.feldenkrais-method.org

Iyengar Yoga: National Association
  of the United States
3010 Hennepin Avenue S #272
Minneapolis, Minnesota 55408
800-889-YOGA
www.iynaus.org

Kripalu Center for Yoga & Health
P.O. Box 793
West Street, Route 183
Lenox, Massachusetts 01240
www.kripalu.org

MayoClinic.com
www.mayoclinic.com/health/back-
  pain/HQ00955

National Institutes of Health
www.nih.gov/od/ors/ds/ergonomics/
  backstrength.html

Occupational Safety and Health
  Administration
www.osha.gov/SLTC/etools/compu
  terworkstations

Pilates Method Alliance
P.O. Box 370906
Miami, Florida 33137-0906
866-573-4945 or 305-573-4946
Fax: 305-573-4461
www.pilatesmethodalliance.org